D0483863

UNDERSTANDING HEPATITIS

Also by Naheed Ali

Understanding Fibromyalgia: An Introduction for Patients and Caregivers

Understanding Chronic Fatigue Syndrome: An Introduction for Patients and Caregivers

Understanding Lung Cancer: An Introduction for Patients and Caregivers

Understanding Celiac Disease: An Introduction for Patients and Caregivers

Understanding Alzheimer's: An Introduction for Patients and Caregivers

Understanding Parkinson's Disease: An Introduction for Patients and Caregivers

The Obesity Reality: A Comprehensive Approach to a Growing Problem

Arthritis and You: A Comprehensive Digest for Patients and Caregivers

Diabetes and You: A Comprehensive, Holistic Approach

UNDERSTANDING HEPATITIS

An Introduction for Patients and Caregivers

Naheed Ali

ROWMAN & LITTLEFIELD
Lanham • Boulder • New York • London

Published by Rowman & Littlefield
An imprint of The Rowman & Littlefield Publishing Group, Inc.
4501 Forbes Boulevard, Suite 200, Lanham, Maryland 20706
www.rowman.com

Unit A, Whitacre Mews, 26-34 Stannary Street, London SE11 4AB

British Library Cataloguing in Publication Information Available

Library of Congress Cataloging-in-Publication Data

Names: Ali, Naheed, 1981- author.
Title: Understanding hepatitis : an introduction for patients and caregivers / Naheed Ali.
Description: Lanham : Rowman & Littlefield, [2018] | Includes bibliographical references and index.
Identifiers: LCCN 2018019972 (print) | LCCN 2018022027 (ebook) | ISBN 9781538117255 (Electronic) | ISBN 9781538117248 (cloth : alk. paper)
Subjects: | MESH: Hepatitis—etiology | Hepatitis—complications | Liver Diseases | Caregivers | Popular Works
Classification: LCC RC848.H425 (ebook) | LCC RC848.H425 (print) | NLM WI 715 | DDC 616.3/623—dc23
LC record available at https://lccn.loc.gov/2018019972

∞ ™ The paper used in this publication meets the minimum requirements of American National Standard for Information Sciences Permanence of Paper for Printed Library Materials, ANSI/NISO Z39.48-1992.

Printed in the United States of America

Understanding Hepatitis is dedicated to my readers, to hepatitis sufferers, and to all who provided encouragement and support for my research.

CONTENTS

III: MANY FACES OF HEPATITIS

IV: RESOLUTIONS

V: HOMESTRETCH

AUTHOR'S NOTE

This book is not meant for medical professionals; however, the non-medical reader may encounter advanced medical terminology throughout the writing. This is often necessary for the intended comprehensive review of the subject and because certain medical concepts necessitate clarification well beyond a modest introduction. A glossary has been placed near the back of the book to explain complex lexicon to those unfamiliar with the language of medicine.

PREFACE

Hepatitis is a disease centered around the inflammation of the liver. The term *hepatitis* is a rather general one and can include illnesses caused by many different sources. Five virus strains have been identified: A, B, C, D, and E viruses. Hepatitis is often induced by toxic substances such as alcohol and certain drugs, autoimmune diseases, the accumulation of fat in the liver, and other rare ailments.[1]

To understand how hepatitis affects the whole body, this book first examines the basics of how it affects the liver. The liver is the largest organ of the human body, apart from the skin, and performs many important functions. The hepatic globules in the liver filter all the blood in the body, eliminating harmful substances, removing both bacteria and worn-out blood cells, as well as forming clotting factors to control bleeding. After a meal, the liver stores nutrients to provide energy. The liver also produces bile, a substance that aids the digestive process in the small intestine. When the hepatitis virus enters the liver, it invades the liver cells and replicates itself. In response, the body directs immune cells to attack both the virus and the liver cells infected with the virus. These liver cells become inflamed and ultimately die. Over time, scar tissue forms around dead and infected liver cells, preventing the liver from working properly.[2]

Depending on the length of the condition, hepatitis can be characterized as acute (lasting less than six months) or chronic (lasting for six months or even for life). Viral hepatitis A and E are acute, while B, C, and D can be chronic. A person with a chronic hepatitis infection has a large amount of scar tissue (a sign of cirrhosis) on the liver, which limits blood flow and shrinks and hardens the liver.[3]

IMPORTANCE OF READING ABOUT HEPATITIS

The number of reported cases of viral hepatitis is shockingly high: 1.4 million infections yearly, and that is for the hepatitis A virus alone. However, a large number of persons with hepatitis remain undiagnosed, meaning that the total number is actually significantly higher. In fact, the World Health Organization (WHO) estimates that approximately 2 billion people have been infected with the hepatitis B virus and more than 400 million people today suffer from chronic hepatitis B or C. The disease is more prevalent in developing countries, where systematic and timely vaccination is more difficult to achieve and densely populated communities can quickly become hotbeds for infection.[4]

Considering how extensive hepatitis is, as well as the large number of deaths it causes, there is surprisingly very little awareness of this disease. Governments often neglect educating the public about how viral hepatitis can be prevented and treated, compared to other fatal viruses like HIV, despite similar numbers of annual victims. As much as nongovernmental organizations work to address this, it remains essential for society to be informed for their own and their family's protection.[5]

The biggest reason hepatitis remains hidden from public consciousness is that frequently its symptoms are unapparent; individuals can be infected with the virus for years and not realize it. This, however, gives the virus time to do its damage and greatly increases the risk of cirrhosis and liver cancer. In such cases, a liver transplant may be necessary, and death becomes a real possibility. It also means that the risk of infecting others greatly increases. This is why proper hepatitis education is important.[6]

The symptoms of hepatitis commonly include loss of appetite, fatigue, muscle or joint aches, fever, nausea, vomiting, and abdominal pain. It is easy to see how these symptoms can be mistaken for the flu or other illnesses. A fever or belly ache does not immediately point to hepatitis, and people generally think little beyond immediate care and pain relief. There is one symptom that is usually linked to hepatitis: yellowing of the skin, also known as jaundice. Although most people associate it with liver disease, there is the assumption that all hepatitis patients develop jaundice, which is not the case. Jaundice does not appear frequently, but when it does, it means that there is already severe liver damage.[7]

Hepatitis A is usually associated with insufficient hygiene practices. The virus is found in the feces of those infected, and the illness is most often transferred through contaminated water or food. The virus can survive for months at room temperature. Infection is common in children in developing countries (nearly 100 percent become infected), but following infection, these children are immune indefinitely.[8]

Patients and caregivers should also know that, in the case of the hepatitis B, C, and D, viruses are transmitted through exposure to infected bodily fluids, most commonly blood. This can occur with sexual contact, transfusions with infected blood, contaminated medical equipment, drug use, tattooing, or body piercing. The virus can live on such household objects as razors or toothbrushes. It is also commonly transmitted from infected mothers to infants at the time of birth. The hepatitis D virus only infects those who already have hepatitis B.[9]

Similar to hepatitis A, hepatitis E is found in contaminated food and water. It is most common in hot climates and is also spread by eating raw shellfish that have come from water contaminated by sewage.[10]

In most cases, hepatitis is self-limiting. Treatment consists mainly of maintaining comfort and healthy nutrition. In the case of chronic illness, however, there are certain drugs, such as interferon and ribavirin, that are effective. Unfortunately, interferon is not widely available globally, and not all patients respond well to it.[11]

A COMPREHENSIVE APPROACH IS VITAL

To counter hepatitis, there must be multiple avenues of attack. First, the public must be educated about hepatitis and how to stay protected. To raise awareness, World Hepatitis Day was instituted on July 28, 2010. In 2014, more than one hundred countries participated in programs around the world. By fostering awareness among people and improving living conditions, nutrition, vaccination, and treatment, hepatitis can be brought under control and possibly even eradicated.[12]

1

Basic Picture

1

INTRODUCTION: IMPORTANCE OF LIVER HEALTH

It has been accepted that one could look younger and healthier as well as extend life span by paying attention to one small thing—the liver. To be precise, the liver is not a small organ in size or impact. Weighing in at an impressive 1.5 kilograms, the liver is a large vital organ necessary to stay alive. This unsung hero is often forgotten due to its background functionality. Even when suffering the occasional damage, it has the ability to repair itself before anything wrong is noticed. It does not beat faster when agitated, like a heart, or rumble when it requires food, like a stomach. However, this behind-the-scenes worker is responsible for performing more than five hundred different functions, in addition to aiding other organs with their own primary tasks.[1]

The liver has been referred to as a control station sitting in the middle of the abdomen. This dark red, wedge-shaped organ processes everything ingested: the gases breathed in, the food eaten, and anything absorbed through the skin. It carefully detoxifies the body by removing waste and sends nutrients to where they are required, in the form required, and at the time required. It keeps the body chugging along efficiently, provides sufficient energy, and helps to fight infections. In the end, the liver is responsible for overall health.[2]

The role of the liver can be apportioned into different functions. All of the blood in the human body is eventually metabolized through the cells in the liver. At any given point, this organ holds a massive amount of the blood. Nutrients from food enter the blood and are either released when required or stored for when the body needs a boost in the future. For instance, when there is shortage of energy, the liver churns out glycogen, a form of glucose processed from the carbohydrates eaten. The liver also creates glycogen from amino acids and other nonsugar sources. It breaks down fat and compounds, including cholesterol, stockpiling them as fat in the cells just beneath the skin. It deploys these fatty reserves as energy to ensure consistent energy levels. Additionally, the liver stores vitamins, including A, B_{12}, D, E, and K, as well as minerals (such as iron and copper) and releases them when the body needs them.[3]

At the same time, the liver is apt enough not to store anything that could harm the body. One of its primary functions is to eliminate toxic substances. It is in charge of secreting a thick green-yellow digestive juice called bile. Until needed to help eliminate waste in the intestine, the bile is simply stored in the gallbladder (it also helps the liver break down fats efficiently). Naturally occurring waste products and harmful toxins from drugs and alcohol are rapidly transported to the intestines or kidneys. They are then swilled out of the system. The liver also extracts nitrogen from proteins, separating the ammonia to be shuttled out of the body in the form of urine.[4]

HOW THE LIVER CONTRIBUTES TO THE SUSTENANCE OF LIFE

The liver plays a big part in the recovery from injuries and illnesses. For instance, it produces the proteins responsible for blood clotting. Without these macronutrients (in this case, proteins), a small cut or bruise would bleed for much longer. When medicines are taken, it is the liver that is in charge of breaking down the active ingredients in them for the body to absorb. It also filters dead cells and harmful bacteria from the blood, further boosting resistance. Hormones are made and broken down by the liver to help regulate blood sugar. In short, it keeps the body strong and ticking.[5]

As society continues to grow increasingly health conscious, information about maintaining safe cholesterol levels and safeguarding against heart disease is widely sought. Yet, the organ working in the background to maintain vital function tends to be ignored. The reality is that the human body cannot survive for more than a day without the liver.[6]

The liver is often overworked in those with indulgent lifestyles. While it is a hardy organ that can even regenerate itself if a part is damaged or removed, it can occasionally shut down, causing serious malfunction within the body.[7] For instance, the bloodstream starts accumulating impurities and the liver is no longer capable of flushing them out. Sugar metabolism levels are no longer regulated, causing coordination problems, sleep disturbances, anxiety, and more. Hormones regulating energy and mood are also affected, not to mention those influencing menstruation and menopause. This in turn makes it burdensome on the body to recover from even small bruises.[8]

HOW LIVER CELLS ADD TO THE HEALTH OF OTHER ORGANS

The liver supports nearly every organ in the body and is indispensable. Without the liver, the digestive system falters, hindering nutrients from being channeled prooperly. The kidneys, which rely on the liver to filter plasma and electrolytes, suddenly create greater quantities of urine, leading to dehydration. Fluid may accumulate within the abdomen, and new veins may form in the stomach as the body reacts to these deviations.[9]

One of the main utilities of the liver is to regulate blood flow. It pumps about 1.4 liters of blood every minute. When this blood flow starts to fail, other organs follow. A shortage of blood flow damages both organs and tissues and could lead to heart failure as the body struggles to cope with an irregular heartbeat.[10]

Studies show the brain is also affected by liver malfunction. Damaged liver cells allow too many toxic substances to travel toward the brain. Unprotected and vulnerable, the brain becomes severely damaged, to the point where it cannot recover. This can be fatal and send the body into coma.[11]

There are several bacteria and viruses that can directly affect the liver, causing illnesses like hepatitis, where the liver becomes inflamed. Hepatitis is usually caused by a virus, and 20 percent of people worldwide are believed to be infected with a hepatitis virus. In the United States, hepatitis A, B, and C are the most common types.[12]

ANALYSIS

Fortunately, the liver is extremely resilient and often recoils back to health with medical intervention. However, it is important to note that lifestyle choices often influence how well the liver functions. It is important to maintain a healthy body mass index (BMI) and stay physically fit. Limiting alcohol intake and being careful with the substances put into the body can also help. Small steps can safeguard the liver and protect it for a lifetime. Liver maintenance truly is one of the most cost-efficient insurance policies anyone could have.[13]

2

ANATOMY OF HEPATITIS

Anatomy is the study of the structure of organisms, from the smallest cell to the largest organ. Anatomy has a sister discipline, physiology, which investigates how these parts work. Of course, function and form are strongly related and complement one another, but the sheer amount of information involved in both necessitates separate study. An intangible disease like hepatitis cannot possess any anatomy. Therefore, this chapter examines how the physical anatomy of a person relates to material issues of the liver.[1]

HUMAN ANATOMY

In the configurations of living organisms, there is a hierarchy of organizations. To start, the human body houses the smallest unit of life, the cell. Cells are made of atoms, about 100 trillion of them for each cell that vary widely in size and shape, depending on their purpose. When similar cells perform a specific function together, they form tissue. The study of cells (cytology) and tissues (histology) forms the tributary of microscopic anatomy. In contrast, macroscopic anatomy, or gross anatomy, refers to body parts that can be studied with the unaided eye. When two or more tissue types combine, they form organs that accomplish important tasks. These organs are grouped together into organ systems. The highest level of anatomical organization is the body itself, scientifically recognized as the *organism*. For a sense of scale, the human body is estimated to contain anywhere from 10 trillion to 70 trillion cells, depending on the measuring scheme used.[2]

Human anatomy has been the object of thousands of years of study. The word *anatomy* comes from the Greek and translates as "to cut open." Over the centuries, anatomy was usually studied through the practice of dissection, which fell out of favor in the Middle Ages due to religious persecution but was reinstated as a way of learning about the human body during the Renaissance. Public dismemberments of corpses were very popular, attended by such artists as Michelangelo and Rembrandt. Leonardo da Vinci used the knowledge gained from dissections extensively in his art and research. During the eighteenth and nineteenth centuries, more and more medical schools were established. Today, students are still taught anatomy using educational cadavers, along with advanced techniques like microscopy, MRIs, and ultrasound imaging. Of course, with technological improvements, other advances were made. Microscopy allows the study of organisms in extreme detail, and MRIs, ultrasound imaging, and other techniques allow subjects to be studied without causing any harm. These technologies are used to diagnose afflictions much more accurately and afford therapeutic services.[3]

ANATOMY OF THE LIVER

For anyone affected by liver disease or hepatitis, it is important to be familiar with the internal composition of the organ. First, one must know where in the body it is located, making it less likely to mistake liver pain for other abdominal issues. Quite often, liver disease goes undiagnosed because its symptoms are easily overlooked. The liver is triangular and extends across almost the entire abdomen, with the bulk of it occupying the upper-right quadrant of the abdomen, immediately below the diaphragm and shielded by the rib cage. It sits on top of the right kidney and the intestines, with the stomach to its left. A type of connective tissue called the peritoneum covers the entire liver and supports and holds it in place. When inflamed, as in hepatitis patients, the liver extends further down toward the midriff and across the upper abdomen.[4]

The bulk of the cells in the liver are hepatocytes. They make up around 80 percent of its volume and are involved in most of the five hundred functions of the liver, including storing and synthesizing proteins and cholesterol, processing carbohydrates, detoxifying blood, and secreting bile. Hepatocytes are roughly hexagonal in shape and stack on top of each other. Millions of hepatocytes together form a hepatic lobule, and there are thousands of these lobules in the liver, each around a central vein that carries blood to the larger hepatic vein and out of the liver. These lobules make up most of the mass of the liver.[5]

The liver is divided into four lobes: the right, left, caudate, and quadrate lobes. The right lobe is by far the largest, separated from the left with a falciform ligament, another type of connective tissue. Liver sinusoids—small blood vessels made up of sinusoidal endothelial cells and large white blood cells called Kupffer cells—are distributed throughout the lobes to carry fluids to and from the cells. Kupffer cells can fight off many bacteria before dying out themselves. Secreted bile is carried out through bile canaliculi that group together into bile ducts.[6]

Other cells in the liver are hepatic stellate cells, affixed in the so-named space of Disse among hepatocytes and liver sinusoids. When the liver of a longtime sufferer of hepatitis develops cirrhosis, the normally soft tissue made up of hepatocytes is swapped for scar tissue made up of hepatic stellate cells. In a healthy liver, the functionality of these cells is still unclear, though they do store vitamin A. However, in the case of liver damage, stellate cells become active and multiply quickly, leading to scar tissue formation. The functionality of the liver then is severely limited, and this crucial organ hardens and shrinks.[7]

The liver is known as the "factory of the body" and is a truly magnificent piece of equipment to have. With the extensive network of blood vessels in the liver, it is clear that maintaining a healthy cardiovascular system is beneficial. The best way to accomplish this is through regular exercise. Because of its importance, the liver is the second-most transplanted organ after the kidney. For hepatitis sufferers, a liver transplant may be necessary, but postsurgical survival rates are rather promising.[8]

ANALYSIS

Anatomy is one of the primogenital branches of science, and every medical student today must have an excellent grasp of it. It is important not only for future physicians and caregivers but also for professionals in areas of fitness, psychology, and law. No matter what people do, they should have a good understanding of their liver. That way, when anything goes wrong with it, caregivers and patients can enlist a trained doctor and handle problems in the best way possible.[9]

3

PHYSIOLOGY OF HEPATITIS

The obvious goal of every organism is to stay alive. To accomplish this, all parts of an organism have to work together and be functional. The science that studies what exactly body parts, from cells to whole humans, do and how they do it is called physiology. It tackles a wide variety of precise questions and answers the big questions, like, How are people alive? and What does it mean to die?[1]

THE IMPORTANCE OF PHYSIOLOGY

In order to comprehend what an organism does, patients and caregivers should understand functions from a scientific standpoint. Hepatitis experts tend to approach physiology and anatomy in tandem because function and structure are complementary. In physiology, everything is connected. No cell, tissue, or organ ever works in isolation, and in fact the interactions of body parts are the key to their setup. The expression "more than the sum of its parts" fits perfectly here.[2]

The ancient Greeks Hippocrates, Aristotle, and Galenus are the founders of human physiology. Hippocrates is of course known as the father of medicine, while Aristotle emphasized the relation between structure and function. Galenus performed many experiments on the operations of the liver, and his theories remained essential in the medical field for more than a thousand years. Two important breakthroughs came in the nineteenth century: first, cell theory, which was revolutionary at the time, and second, the concept of homeostasis. Since then, physiology has developed exponentially due to technological advancements.[3]

Homeostasis, meaning "balance and stability," is a property of all living beings. The prolonged loss of homeostasis inevitably leads to death. Internal homeostasis of the human body means that chemical processes and substances, such temperature, acidity, oxygen, blood glucose, and water, must be kept within specific limits at all times. The way this is accomplished is usually through a negative feedback loop, a process that requires three elements: a receptor, a control center, and an effector. When a receptor detects a certain imbalance in an organ, such as the liver, it sends the information to the control center, often the hypothalamus in the brain. The control center then instructs effectors to regulate the situation until the receptors no longer detect an anomaly. Homeostasis is experiential when it comes to everyday life: When the body get too warm, it starts sweating to decrease body temperature, and when it is cold, the muscles shiver to increase it. Even the feeling of thirst is a homeostatic response to elevated salt levels in the bloodstream. Regarding salt levels, the liver works in conjunction with the kidneys because of excessive sodium buildup in hepatitis patients.[4]

Aside from its importance for students in the medical field, knowledge of physiology is certainly helpful for those hepatitis sufferers struggling to lose weight. When the body is deprived of food, it resets the normal metabolic rate to a level lower than usual. This allows one to function even while starving, albeit not as well. Thus, eating less might cause one to lose weight in the beginning, but after metabolism adjusts, this loss stops. The solution is to force the metabolism to function at a higher rate through physical exercise and exhaust reserve energy stores. When everything is running smoothly, the many constant operations within cannot be noticed by others. It is when something goes wrong—when the patient feels pain—that knowledge of physiology is needed.[5]

Pathophysiology, an offshoot of physiology, is concerned with how the normal functioning of the body is affected by illness. Hepatitis patients can help their bodies fight the disease by being well versed in pathophysiology, putting themselves in the best position to succeed. Knowing about the detoxification process in the liver makes it clear why alcohol ingestion is unhealthy, especially for hepatitis patients. Because the liver already performs so many functions, when it also has to fight hepatitis, it takes on a lot of stress. By eating healthy foods that need minimal processing, one allows the liver to devote more of its resources to tackling the virus.[6]

SPECIFIC PHYSIOLOGY OF THE LIVER

The liver performs more than five hundred functions in the body, cooperating with many other organs and organ systems. A lot of blood flows through the liver from two main sources: the hepatic artery brings oxygenated blood from the heart, and the hepatic portal vein brings nutrient-rich blood from the digestive system. When blood leaves the liver, it does so through central veins located in every hepatic lobule that join together into the larger hepatic veins.[7]

Besides serving as an organ, the liver is considered a gland because it exudes bile. This substance leaves the hepatic lobules through hepatic ducts and is stored in the gallbladder, ready to be used. As eaten food reaches the duodenum, bile is gushed through the common bile duct to help emulsify fats, neutralize extra stomach acids, and remove such waste products as bilirubin.[8]

The liver sorts out some of the nutrients brought in from the digestive system. Depending on such physiological factors as the level of blood glucose, the pancreas secretes hormones that tell the liver how to process incoming glucose from food. If levels are too high, then glucose is converted into glycogen and stored for later use. Otherwise, it is regularly dispatched back into the bloodstream. When glucose levels drop too low, the stored glycogen is converted to glucose for use. Aside from glycogen, a number of vitamins and minerals are stored in the liver, with some reserves large enough to last more than a year. This storage allows the body to maintain homeostasis even in dire circumstances.[9]

The liver also synthesizes such lipids as cholesterol, which are an important part of cell membranes. Lipids are repetitively recycled internally as an energy source. Amino acids are used to synthesize different proteins acting as blood-clotting factors, as well as albumin, which regulates the water level in blood. If needed, they can also be turned into glucose for energy. Blood flowing into the liver does not contain only nutrients. Alcohol and drugs are also metabolized into less harmful substances, and excess hormones secreted by other glands also broken down. The liver turns ammonia resulting from the processing of amino acid into the less-toxic urea, which is rid from the body through urine. Kupffer cells lining the blood vessels in the liver capture and destroy bacteria, debris, and worn-out red blood cells. Millions of red blood cells are disposed of every minute.[10]

ANALYSIS

In the legend, Prometheus gifted fire to humanity. Zeus punished him by chaining him to a rock, where his liver was consumed by a bird of prey every day, only to grow back nightly. A fitting if extreme allegory for the resilient powerhouse known as the liver.[11]

Physiologically, the liver differs from other internal organs in an intriguing way: It is capable of naturally regenerating damaged tissue. Liver cells are often affected by confronting harmful toxins and bacteria, but as little as 25 percent of a liver can self-repair into a full-sized organ. Hepatocytes are largely undifferentiated throughout the liver's mass, so they reenter the cell division cycle and multiply. Thus, even extensive liver damage can be overturned, allowing the patient to resume regular functioning. This remarkable ability is particularly useful during liver transplant operations.[12]

4

DIGESTIVE HEALTH

The body cannot do much with bread, meat, and fruit in their natural state. This is where the digestive system comes in. It is tasked with extracting nutrients from the food we eat and removing the waste from the body. These nutrients give everyone, especially hepatitis patients, energy to function.[1]

After food has been chewed and enzymes in the saliva have worked their magic, it becomes a bolus that is swallowed. The bolus travels through the rest of the system, thanks to muscle contractions called peristalsis. After going down the esophagus and landing in the stomach, the gastric juices (a mix of hydrochloric acid and pepsin) break down the bolus into a pasty substance called chyme. Chyme enters the first section of the small intestine (which is actually quite large, up to 10.5 meters long), called the duodenum. Here, enzymes from the pancreas and bile made by the liver and stored in the gallbladder mix with the chyme; the rest of the small intestine has the vital job of absorbing the released nutrients and getting them into the bloodstream. All of the remaining mass then goes from the small intestine to the large intestine, where water is absorbed and the waste is ready to be eliminated.[2]

HOW THE DIGESTIVE TRACT SUSTAINS LIFE

The digestive system contains a vast portion of the body's immune system and harvests most of the body's serotonin, a neurotransmitter thought to help regulate mood or emotions. Poor overall digestive system health is connected to sicknesses in other organ systems, including the immune system. Stress can exacerbate the symptoms of digestive illnesses, such as queasiness, bloating, irritable bowel syndrome, and inflammatory bowel syndrome. An unhealthy diet rich in fat and sugar puts strain on the digestive system, forcing it to work harder and longer to process meals; the stomach then produces more acid, which can lead to ulcers, gastric reflux, and other issues. Healthy digestion cannot work in the absence of water, and proper hydration provides the essential amount of moisture for the digestive system to function.[3]

There are numerous other afflictions of the gastrointestinal (GI) tract: abdominal pain, blood in the stool, bloating, constipation, diarrhea, incontinence, heartburn, nausea, vomiting, and difficulty swallowing. Disease, stress, lack of sleep, and such medications as antibiotics can disturb the delicate balance of good and bad bacteria in the digestive tract. Excessive bad bacteria may manifest in painful digestive symptoms or serious infections.[4]

Considering the fact that the liver alone performs hundreds of important functions in collaboration with most of the human body's systems, it is clear why its job must be made as easy as possible, especially for hepatitis patients. To ease the burden on the liver, the entire digestive system must function efficiently. The best natural way to accomplish this is through carefully managed nutrition. A poor diet worsens the liver's problems. Overeating causes excess fat to build up in the liver and leads to fatty liver, which increases the risk of cirrhosis and diminishes the efficiency of drugs to treat hepatitis. Hepatitis sufferers who consume more alcohol than the liver can handle hasten the progression of the disease, leading to more complications over time.[5]

From a holistic perspective, there are some basic guidelines for defeating hepatitis. A good rule of thumb is that variation is always better. Plenty of whole-grain breads and cereals provide much-needed carbohydrates. Fruits and vegetables provide antioxidants to fight cell damage and are typically low in fat but rich in vitamins and fiber. Protein found in meat, dairy, and eggs helps to repair or replace damaged liver cells. It is also essential to drink plenty of fluids to replace those lost in fighting hepatitis.[6]

It is generally recommended to eat smaller meal portions more often (at least three times a day) to maintain a high energy level. Remaining energetic is always helpful for otherwise healthy individuals, but hepatitis patients benefit from regular exercise more than usual. A healthy lifestyle staves off fat, improves appetite, and helps the liver in the detoxifying process through sweating. Activity boosts the immune system and reduces the risk of nonalcoholic fatty liver disease and diabetes.[7]

HOW THE DIGESTIVE SYSTEM SUPPORTS OTHER ORGANS

Without the work of the digestive system, the rest of the body could not operate. The liver is a living cleaning station. One of its main tasks is filtering the body's blood. It arrives from two sources: the heart, through the hepatic artery, and blood vessels surrounding the small intestine, through the hepatic portal vein. The nutrients brought by the blood are processed in the hepatic lobules and are then redistributed throughout the body's tissues as needed or stored for future use. To put it simply, no one can function without fuel prepared by the liver.[8]

The blood flowing into the liver carries both nutrients and toxins. The hepatocytes filter these substances out of the blood and make them harmless or propel them through the excretory system to be eliminated. Other unusable byproducts are converted by hepatocytes into bile, which in turn aids general digestion in the small intestine.[9]

The liver also contributes to the cardiovascular organs by constructing blood plasma proteins used in blood clots. Hepatocytes secrete the hormone somatomedin, which promotes cell growth, and manufacture cholesterol needed for the creation of other hormones. Other organs in the digestive system also secrete important hormones. For example, the pancreas produces insulin, which metabolizes fats and carbohydrates.[10]

The GI tract is lined with millions of neurons. They form the enteric nervous system (ENS) and are the origin of the phrase "gut feeling." Because the majority of serotonin in the body is located in the GI tract, a properly functioning digestive system underwrites the general feeling of well-being in healthy humans.[11]

ANALYSIS

It is undeniably clear that the digestive system has a fundamental role in enabling other organs in the body to function properly. Also, crucial nutrients, such as fats, vitamins, and carbohydrates, are carried to the liver, which has the important task of storing them for future use and making glycogen, an energy reserve for the body.[12]

5

CIRCULATORY SYSTEM HEALTH

The heart has been a symbol for the essence of the human body since ancient times. Even ages ago, the importance of the heart was understood in medicine. The 3,500-year-old Ebers Papyrus found in Egypt includes a section that names the heart as the organ responsible for distributing the blood supply to every body part through connected vessels. It is a simple but correct description of the circulatory system. In the modern era, it is known that this system consists of the cardiovascular and lymphatic branches.[1]

THE CARDIOVASCULAR SYSTEM

The cardiovascular system is the most recognizable and is tasked with circulating oxygen and other nutrients, as well as maintaining homeostasis. This system is made up of three main components: the heart, the blood vessels, and the blood itself. The heart pumps blood through blood vessels. Of course, it is not quite as simple as that. The heart needs to be strong in order to keep blood flowing, which is why it is almost completely composed of muscle. When even the tiniest blood vessels are accounted for, there are around thousands of miles of blood vessels that reach every part of the human body. Through this network of vessels, the heart thrusts blood made up of blood plasma and cells. There are three types of blood cells: red blood cells, white blood cells, and the often-neglected platelets. Circulating blood, including through the liver, is a continuous process that cannot be voluntarily halted.[2]

Oxygenated blood is carried out of the heart by the aorta, which splits into arteries, and is driven through the rest of the body. These blood vessels branch off into smaller arterioles and then further into the miniscule-sized capillaries to increase the overall surface area to which oxygen and nutrients are delivered to all cells in a process called diffusion. Capillaries take out waste products such as carbon dioxide, which they carry into veins flowing together to form broader waste units, to where the largest vein enters the heart. The deoxygenated blood is then carried out into another circuit through the pulmonary artery to the lungs, where red blood cells trade the carbon dioxide for fresh oxygen. Through the pulmonary veins, the oxygenated blood flows back into the heart, and this run repeats itself more than a thousand times a day.[3]

The heart needs oxygen and nutrients, too. These are supplied by the coronary arteries. When there is a blockage inside one of those arteries, usually because of the accumulation of surplus fat and cholesterol, the muscles of the heart do not receive the necessary energy to do their job. This is what causes a heart attack, which can lead to death. In the United States, diseases of the cardiovascular system are the foremost cause of death, and ischemic heart disease causes more than 10 percent of deaths worldwide.[4]

The digestive system extracts nutrients from food. Now, these nutrients need to be distributed throughout the circulatory system and the liver to keep cells full of energy. As the nutrients are separated, they pass from the GI tract to the capillaries that surround it. The nutrient-rich blood flows through a group of blood vessels called the hepatic (liver) portal system to the liver. Once the liver has taken care of unwanted toxins, the nutrients are ready to be delivered through hepatic veins. These veins carry the blood back to the heart, beginning the pulmonary cycle for oxygenation and returning to feed new oxygen to all the cells in the body. One can see how the liver depends on the cardiovascular system to complete its tasks. If the liver itself has trouble, as it does for hepatitis patients, the supply of amino acids, vitamins, and other nutrients to the rest of the body is ebbed. This in turn affects the body's ability to efficiently distribute the necessary fuel for normal function.[5]

One of the best methods of strengthening cardiovascular system health is exercise. The heart can atrophy from a lack of physical activity. However, regular exercise helps the hepatitis patient's heart grow stronger. It can be trained to pump more blood and with less effort. Exercise stimulates the growth of new capillaries to feed tissues and makes existing capillaries larger. This makes it easier for all cells to get their supply of energy. As the heart and blood vessels become larger and stronger, the rate at which the heart beats to pump blood can afford to slow down. Thus, while resting, the heart can conserve energy and become less susceptible to organismal problems.[6]

Exercise also increases the volume of blood, and consequently the number of red blood cells, in the body. Thus, more oxygen is transported with each circulatory cycle, and waste products are removed more efficiently. It becomes much harder for fat to accumulate around arteries and other organs, including the liver.[7]

Blood contains a large amount of white blood cells, called leukocytes, that are part of the immune system. For hepatitis patients, leukocytes flood into the liver to handle the damaged cells, as well as the virus, in the case of viral hepatitis. To sustain a faster and larger supply of white blood cells, blood vessels expand, causing inflammation.[8]

THE LYMPHATIC SYSTEM

The lymphatic system is the other, lesser-known part of the circulatory system, but it is just as important. When nutrients from capillaries diffuse to cells, they do so jointly with blood plasma, which fuses with interstitial fluid (the fluid that surrounds all the cells in the body) and makes this transfer possible. The plasma then picks up waste and toxins, but not all of the plasma makes the trek back into the blood vessels. To pick up this extra fluid, called lymph, there are lymphatic capillaries that carry it to a large network of vessels that pass through lymph nodes. Eventually the lymph reenters the bloodstream through the subclavian veins, located near the neck.[9]

Interestingly, the lymphatic system lacks a central pump like the heart to push the lymph—which is twice as abundant as blood—through the body. Instead, lymph is pumped through muscle contractions called peristalsis, similar to how food is thrust through the digestive tract. The lymphatic system's most important feature is the lymph nodes. These small, oval structures filter the lymph for whatever dangerous substances there might be. Lymph contains its own stock of white blood cells called lymphocytes produced by the spleen, the bone marrow, and a special gland known as the thymus. These lymphocytes are abundant in the lymph nodes. They can be separated into T cells and B cells.[10]

When a bacterium is singled out, the lymph nodes make more infection-fighting white blood cells, which can cause swelling. This is why hepatitis sufferers can sometimes feel swollen nodes in their necks or armpits. The white blood cells attack the bacteria and destroy it, while also producing proteins known as antibodies to alert other immune system cells of the problem. T cells also "instruct" other white blood cells to store information about the harmful microbes in case of future attacks.[11]

ANALYSIS

The circulatory system is always toiling away to keep the human body alive and healthy. It is like having a personal cook, gym trainer, and bodyguard all in one. This system, of which the heart is the center, extends throughout the entire individual. It may not have the mystical qualities as people long ago believed, but it does a reasonably good job nonetheless.[12]

6

HISTORY OF HEPATITIS

The history of medicine is chock-full with superstitions, mistakes, and accidental discoveries. However, it is also full of astonishing insight, tireless research, and courageous experimentation. The science of diagnosing, treating, and preventing illness, such as hepatitis, has a turbulent past, changing immensely since the times of mystical medicine men. Yet, there are medicinal herbs that are still proving useful today, thousands of years after their first use. The theory of the "four humors" now seems silly and unhelpful, but the thought that four bodily fluids determined the health of every individual still had mainstream supporters well into the nineteenth century, even after the invention of the microscope and the discovery of the cell.[1]

The Hippocratic oath is well over two millennia old, and yet doctors today still follow this code of ethics. Galen's historical studies were remarkable but fraught with errors, and it took another thousand years before the hand of religion loosened its grip on the human body enough to allow Renaissance-era physician Andreas Vesalius to write his own crucial works on the liver. Vesalius attended the University of Pavia in Italy, and by then, Western Europe had adopted the model of the first medical schools from those in the Middle East. Medicine was both a science and an art, but it was usually a very bloody combination of the two in the literal sense. Surgery was often brutal, with little survival expectancy, and was in fact performed not by doctors, who considered it beneath them, but by barbers. Ambrose Paré was one such barber-surgeon who performed surgeries with groundbreaking techniques on sixteenth-century battlefields. Now he is considered the father of modern surgery. Necessity is the mother of invention, and what task is more rallying than saving lives?[2]

Edward Jenner always put his faith in research and experiments: He vaccinated his gardener's eight-year-old son against smallpox in 1796. This sparked the single-most effective method of preventing disease today. The last two hundred years have brought more breakthroughs than one could have imagined: pasteurization, X-rays, penicillin, DNA, and organ transplants, to name just a few. It is owing to exceptional people and their amazing discoveries that advances in hepatology have come this far. Many (though sadly not all) people can now expect to live their lives seriously unmarred by disease.[3]

HISTORY OF LIVER DISEASES

Sicknesses of the liver have been studied since the dawn of modern medicine, and cancers (liver cancer is the second-highest cause of deaths) have been referenced in scrolls dating back to ancient Egypt. Hippocrates named the disease *cancer* because the striations in malignant tumors look similar to a crab's feet.[4] He also wrote about jaundice, or icterus, and linked it to the liver. He recognized the hardening of the liver as a symptom of disease. Greek anatomist Galen considered the liver to be the central organ of the human body, while Aretaeus of Cappadocia theorized jaundice to be caused by the spilling of bile, manufactured by the liver, into the bloodstream.[5]

In more recent times, nineteenth-century physician Victor Hanot made numerous advances in the field of hepatology. He researched many liver diseases and primary biliary cirrhosis, also referred to as Hanot's disease, which affects the bile ducts, causes the accumulation of bile, and damages tissues, leading to cirrhosis. The first human liver transplant was conducted in 1963, an operation performed by Thomas Starzl.[6]

HISTORY OF HEPATITIS

Records of jaundice epidemics in ancient China and Mesopotamia, as well as during the Roman Empire, point to probable instances of viral hepatitis outbreaks. The term *hepatitis* was first used in the eighteenth century and is derived from the Greek word *hepar*, meaning "liver," and *-itis*, meaning "inflammation." Hepatitis was commonplace during wartime, for example during the American Civil War and World War II. Tens of thousands of hepatitis cases were identified in the first war, though the number of infections in the latter case is estimated to be around 16 million. An outbreak in 1942 following yellow fever vaccines led Frederic MacCallum to theorize the existence of two different hepatitis viruses: type A, or infectious hepatitis, characterized by a transitory incubation period, and type B, or serum hepatitis, which has a longer incubation period. Regulations blocking blood donors with a background marked by hepatitis began in the late 1950s—long before the identification of hepatitis viruses or the use of screening tests.[7]

The most important breakthrough came in 1963. Dr. Baruch Blumberg was conducting research on the susceptibility to disease of various aboriginal populations. In the blood sample of an Australian aborigine, he identified a nameless antigen, later labeled the Australia antigen. Following additional investigation, it was determined that the antigen detected the presence of the hepatitis B virus in the blood. This led to another momentous invention in 1981, the hepatitis B vaccine. It was the first vaccine prepared from blood plasma instead of tissue culture and was called the anticancer vaccine because the hepatitis B virus is a common cause of liver cancer.[8]

In 1977, a new antigen was discovered during tests on hepatitis B patients. This led to the identification of the hepatitis D virus. This is the smallest human virus identified thus far and is extremely contagious. This virus requires the host to be already infected with hepatitis B, but it can be prevented through vaccine.[9]

Although hepatitis A, or short-incubation hepatitis, was known to be separate from the other viruses and transmitted through contaminated food and water, not blood, the virus itself was only identified in the late 1970s. A successful vaccine was brought to the table in 1992.[10]

Prior to 1989, the hepatitis C virus was referred to as non-A, non-B virus because the specific agent could not be detected, even though the illness it caused was recognized. The identification of the virus was made through a pioneering, direct molecular approach that paved the way for the discovery of many other previously unknown viruses. Unfortunately, a vaccine for hepatitis C has yet to be developed, and it remains one of the leading culprits of hepatic cancer. The path to a cure however is near with the development and implementation of screening methods for transmission.[11]

The final piece of the hepatitis puzzle was discovered in 1983: the hepatitis E virus. Although transmitted in the same manner as hepatitis A, interestingly it can also be found in domestic animals, such as pigs. A vaccine was produced in China and was approved for use in 2012.[12]

ANALYSIS

There is a tremendous benefit for hepatitis patients to have a familiarity with the history of medicine. It allows society to (1) appreciate how far human civilization has come, (2) recognize the virtue of those brilliant people who went against the grain by using the scientific method, and (3) save untold lives and alleviate the pain of many others.[13]

7

GLOBAL SCALE OF HEPATITIS

Advances in medical technology like the microscope helped put the miasma theory, the theory that breathing in bad air caused diseases like cholera, to bed and gave physicians and researchers a renewed determination to study the causes, patterns, and effects of diseases affecting populations. This work is now called epidemiology.[1]

John Snow was one such physician whose work proved crucial in the then-emerging scientific field. In 1854, there was an outbreak of cholera in London. Snow rejected the miasma theory and set out to find the true source of the epidemic by making use of statistics and geographic distribution. He figured out that contaminated water from a single pump was used by the majority of those infected and was causing a wide array of illnesses, such as hepatitis. The discovery had an immense effect on public health and is recognized as a watershed case for the importance of epidemiology at large.[2]

The most prominent recent case of infectious disease in the Western world has been HIV/AIDS. It was first publicized in 1981 in the United States, although it had been unidentified for decades. The stigma of the disease had great cultural impact, and the effect on public health was even greater. It led to a population-wide acceptance of condom use, a voluntary, individual method of disease prevention on a global scale.[3]

A new branch of medical science, molecular pathological epidemiology, has been gaining importance and was made possible through state-of-the-art technology. It illuminates the etiology (the cause) of disease at molecular, individual, and population levels synchronously.[4]

Epidemiology is used by all health-care workers, regardless of their specialization. It is also useful for everyone else, as the HIV/AIDS case showed. Public health statistics have led to safer working environments, promotion of healthier consumables, and recognition of the effects of abusing such substances as tobacco and alcohol. Demographics of health are used tangentially as a measure of a country's progress; tourists can use this information to understand possible risk factors and methods of disease prevention. Handwashing after using the bathroom and before touching food is now a ubiquitous habit due to the awareness of it as prevention of hepatitis A and E infections and many other diseases.[5]

HEPATITIS: A PANDEMIC, NOT AN EPIDEMIC

When referring to problems hepatitis patients experience, many different terms are used. Some are more precise than others, and some imply a value judgment. Hepatitis is usually referred to as a *condition*, *disorder*, *illness*, or *disease*. A medical *condition* refers to the state of a person, usually when he or she does not function typically. It is a general term often used to refer to the degree to which someone is affected, such as "stable condition" or "critical condition." *Disorder* is similarly broad in definition and expresses a neutral viewpoint. It can refer to physical, mental, or emotional afflictions. The term *illness* implies a poor state of being, though with possibly indeterminate causes. For a more precise description, the term *disease* is applied. It refers to physical impairment, whether infectious or not, and frequently has recognizable causes and symptoms. All these terms can be applied to hepatitis and are sometimes used interchangeably. In medical settings, the word *disease* is preferred.[6]

Hepatitis is without doubt a pandemic. Infections have been reported in every country and practically every part of the world. The rate of infection and the number of deaths has increased steadily over time. More than 500 million people worldwide are infected with hepatitis, and new outbreaks occur often, particularly in developing countries. More than half of even developed countries like the EU have poor to nonexistent data on diseases like Hepatitis C.[7]

WORLDWIDE STATISTICS OF HEPATITIS

New hepatitis A infections affect 1.4 million people yearly. In 1988, tainted seafood caused an outbreak of hepatitis A in Shanghai and affected more than 300,000 people. Small, tight-knit communities and villages can quickly become infected if the main water or food source is contaminated. More than 400 million people are chronically infected with hepatitis B or C. A vaccine against hepatitis C remains one of medicine's greatest and most important challenges.[8]

Hepatitis B affects the most people, an estimated 350 million. Around 20 percent of those will develop cirrhosis or liver cancer during their lives. It is endemic in certain countries. For example, a third of hepatitis B–infected people live in China, 40 million in India, and 12 million in Indonesia. A significant contribution to the prevalence in certain populations is transmission from mother to child during birth. In these regions, child immunization programs are an important focus of public health. Another important factor of transmission is sexual contact. Hepatitis B viruses are much more infectious than the similarly transmitted HIV, with up to one-third of the sexual partners of infected people catching the disease.[9]

A very minute percentage of the world's population is infected with hepatitis C, with more than three million new cases every year. Up to two-thirds of those develop chronic illness. A particularly high rate of infection is in Egypt, with estimates ranging from 15 to more than 20 percent of the population. This has been concomitant with the widespread use of unsterilized equipment during campaigns to treat other diseases, such as schistosomiasis. In high-income lands, most cases of hepatitis C occur in drug users. It is estimated that 90 percent of those who inject drugs and share needles have hepatitis C. The most common cause of transmission is contaminated blood transfusion. Before screening methods were introduced, about 200,000 new cases were reported in the United States yearly. Because the hepatitis D virus cannot spread without the presence of the hepatitis B virus, it is prevalent in the same areas, particularly Africa and South America. Around 5 percent of those with hepatitis B carriers are thought to be coinfected. Hepatitis E has a large prevalence in pregnant women and can develop into a dangerous, often deadly form. Outbreaks occur at a high rate due to contaminated food and water supplies, with around three million acute cases yearly.[10]

The most unfortunate statistic linked to Hepatitis B is the number of deaths. Hepatitis B and C cause 80 percent of liver cancer cases worldwide, which is the second-most dangerous type of cancer. Hepatitis A causes around one hundred deaths yearly in the United States and more than 100,000 globally. The deadliest variety is hepatitis B, responsible for one million deaths annually, or two every minute. It is the tenth-leading cause of death. Five thousand of those deaths occur in the United States. Another 15,000 U.S. patients die from hepatitis C complications, with a total of 350,000 worldwide. As of 2010, 57,000 deaths were caused by hepatitis E every year. In total, an estimated 1.5 million people's deaths are attributed yearly to the various types of viral hepatitis. However, vaccines for hepatitis A, B, and E are 95 to 100 percent efficient, and more than 170 countries around the world organize hepatitis vaccination initiatives for children.[11]

ANALYSIS

The study of the rise of disease in a population has been a cornerstone of public health efforts. Before germs were proven and accepted as the cause of many infectious diseases, folks generally believed that the source of illness was some sort of miasma, or "bad air," that originated from those already infirmed. Luckily, modern technology has allowed for a much more defined approach to the matter.[12]

II

Clinical Picture

8

PATHOLOGY OF HEPATITIS

As physiology tells how organisms work in their normal state, pathology studies how disease disturbs the normal functioning of individuals. The functional impairment is detected through signs and symptoms. Symptoms are felt by the patient, whereas signs are physically observed by someone else. For example, a person with measles may experience tiredness as a symptom, while rashes on the skin noticed by a doctor is a sign. Rashes can be a symptom, too, if the patient observes them, while pain or tiredness cannot be signs because they are intangible. This chapter focuses on the hepatitis patient's signs and symptoms of disease.[1]

Familiarity with the pathology of hepatitis is crucial to recovering normal function. Without knowing how symptoms are related to diseases, people would revert to old pseudoscientific theories, such as the four humors and miasma. If all symptoms are attributed to the same general cause, then treatment methods can be suitably vague and potentially life threatening instead of helpful. The days of bloodletting (drawing blood from the patient) as the all-in-one solution to every ailment are long gone.[2]

HEPATITIS PATHOLOGY

One reason hepatitis is so dangerous is that it can infect the body for years without any observable symptoms. Other times, the symptoms are nonspecific, such as abdominal pain. When one has a belly ache, one doesn't normally think about hepatitis or the liver at all, so the pain might pass after taking an analgesic and sleeping it off, to be forgotten soon thereafter.[3]

Abdominal pain is a common symptom of hepatitis, but there are many more. The signs and symptoms of hepatitis can be divided into three categories: digestive problems, largely caused by reduced bile in the GI tract; physical indicators, such as liver inflammation and tenderness; and other signs and symptoms derived directly from the impairment of hepatic functionality. The incidence and time line of these symptoms are contingent with whether the hepatitis infection is acute (lasting less than six months) or chronic (lasting greater than six months).[4]

ACUTE HEPATITIS

When a person is affected by acute hepatitis, lesions materialize in the liver, thereby marshalling lymphocytes, Kupffer cells, and swollen hepatocytes to the scene. Some tissue necrosis may occur but not usually. Even though the functioning of the liver is affected, its normal architecture is largely undisturbed.[5]

The progression of acute hepatitis is divided into three stages. The first is the pre-icteric stage (*icterus* means "jaundice"). Initial symptoms appear a few weeks after infection and are comparable to flu symptoms, usually digestive in nature. They include general malaise, headache and fever, nausea, loss of appetite, vomiting or diarrhea, and in some cases muscle and joint pain.[6]

Usually within ten days of the first symptoms, jaundice manifests as the yellowing of the skin and eyes. It is launched by the accumulation of bilirubin, normally disposed of in the bile of a healthy liver through the excretory system. Although typically representative of liver damage, jaundice is not synonymous with it, and often appears only in the latter stages of illness. If jaundice does not develop, then the hepatitis is anicteric. At this stage, previous digestive symptoms may subside. Palpable signs include enlargement of the liver and, occasionally, enlargement of lymph nodes. Other signs are dark-colored urine and stool discoloration. Jaundice usually regresses over a period of two weeks, and in the recovery phase, normal liver physiology is reinstated. Feelings of weakness may persist for a month or so, but no long-term damage remains, and immunity for life is a beneficial result.[7]

CHRONIC HEPATITIS

Chronic hepatitis is precarious because the pathology can take a while to decipher. The course of the disease is extremely variable from individual to individual. Tiredness and malaise are possible symptoms, but chronic infections are usually detected through incidental blood tests or screening programs. Jaundice indicates substantial liver damage. Liver inflammation may be detected through physical examination. Signs of long-term chronic hepatitis are weight loss, leg swelling, and fluid accumulation in the abdomen. Because the liver fails to synthesize clotting factors as well, bleeding from injury takes longer to coagulate—an alarming sign. Other signs linked to hepatic function impairment are hyperglycemia, hypoglycemia, and low cholesterol levels.[8]

In up to 20 percent of chronic cases, fibrosis and ultimately cirrhosis develops. Fibrosis is excessive scar tissue that forms in response to hepatocyte injury over an extended period. It damages the structure of the liver and tends to progress toward cirrhosis. Hepatocytes begin multiplying to replace lost ones in isolated groups because space is already appropriated to scar tissue. These isolated groups are called regenerative nodules. The new cells require a blood supply in order to function, but even though new blood vessels form, they are blocked by the fibrotic tissue. This is cirrhosis, a condition that can worsen to the point of total liver failure.[9]

OUTLOOK

The following are the causes of hepatitis[10]:

- **Hepatitis A:** Contaminated food or water.
- **Hepatitis B:** Sexually transmitted through infected blood, semen, or other body fluids.

- **Hepatitis C:** Direct contact with infected blood. Transmission can happen with blood donations from the infected.
- **Hepatitis D:** Only through coinfection with hepatitis B.
- **Hepatitis E:** Water contaminated with the hepatitis E virus.

Each hepatitis strand is caused by a different virus. The most common strands are hepatitis A (HAV), hepatitis B (HBV), and hepatitis C (HCV). HAV is the least dangerous of the three, followed by HBV, which has a chronic form that can lead to such impediments as cirrhosis and even liver failure in extreme cases. With the proper treatment, most patients recover completely from these infections. Nowadays, strong vaccines against HAV and HBV are used, which have significantly decreased the number of cases. However, difficulties arise with HCV because it is asymptomatic and can take years for people to realize they have it. HCV can lead to serious complications, such as liver cancer or liver failure, and unfortunately, there is no vaccine against HCV.[11]

Understanding how the liver is affected by hepatitis helps the patient on the road to rehabilitation. Because an affected liver cannot toil at its normal rate of efficiency, the typical indulgences of life turn dangerous. Drinking alcohol, eating fatty foods, and not exercising puts the affected liver under pressure that can eventually spiral out of control. This is why patients with hepatitis have a controlled diet, including restricting alcohol, and are encouraged to be physically active. Taking care of the body also means that other diseases are less likely to develop concurrently. This allows the immune system to focus as many resources as possible on eliminating the exact source of the pathology, in this case a virus, from the body.[12]

The liver is a remarkable organ: It can regenerate itself to full health even if only a quarter of its mass remains. In some situations, the destruction is too severe and irreversible, resulting in liver failure. Hepatitis can cause liver failure, as well, through such associated conditions as cirrhosis and liver cancer. The only solution, then, would be a liver transplant. Understanding the consequences of pursuing a transplant is vital for making a decision about the future of someone with severe hepatitis.[13]

ANALYSIS

Doctors use signs and symptoms to diagnose patients, while pathologists study the cause, or etiology, of a particular disease. Although no patient wants to face hepatitis, there is good news: In an otherwise healthy adult, there is a high likelihood that treatment can destroy the virus, and the patient can fully recover.[14]

9

RISK FACTORS AND CAUSES

Clarifying the cause of a disease is an important step toward developing an effective treatment and preventing its spread. In order to create vaccines against diseases caused by microorganisms, the infectious organism must first be identified. In medicine, etiology (derived from the Greek word for "reasoning, causality") is the analysis of the causes behind diseases.[1]

The germ theory enriched the whole paradigm of etiology of such diseases as hepatitis. Marcus Terentius Varro, an ancient Roman scholar, wrote something staggering in his tomes on agriculture: One of his characters is told that establishing a farm near a swamp is dangerous because in it live very small creatures, too negligible to see, that float through the air and into the body, causing disease. When he asks how to prevent diseases and whether he should inherit such a farm, he is promptly advised to get rid of the place. About 1,600 years later, in the sixteenth century, the germ theory was first proposed. It was theorized (and proven through three centuries' of research) that microorganisms, invisible to the naked eye, invade a living host, human or otherwise, causing disease.[2]

LIFESTYLE RISK FACTORS OF HEPATITIS

There are a wide range of factors in everyday life that can lead to hepatitis. In all cases, an unhealthy diet is a significant risk factor. Eating too little results in nutrient deficiencies, while overeating leads to obesity or diabetes, making the liver vulnerable. Vitamin deficiencies, excessive lipids in the diet, and a lack of fluids are some specific dangers.[3]

The World Health Organization estimates that, globally, every person aged fifteen and over, consumes 1.6 gallons of pure alcohol annually. Moderate drinking can be handled by the liver in the detoxification process, but with excessive long-term consumption, one can develop alcoholic hepatitis. For men, eighty grams or more of alcohol every day is enough to lead to hepatitis, while for women, half of that amount is dangerous, making them more susceptible to the disease. Around 35 percent of heavy drinkers develop alcoholic hepatitis.[4]

Besides alcohol, the liver must also process such medicines as antibiotics and analgesics. Taking these drugs can cause cell damage and even structural liver damage, leading to toxic hepatitis. It is always better to consult a doctor before taking any medicine, especially if it is in large quantities. Certain dietary supplements and mushroom poisoning can also engender hepatitis in a person. The risk of drug-induced hepatitis grows with age and flourishes with alcohol consumption, as does working in certain environments with exposure to toxic chemicals.[5]

Another form of hepatitis is known as nonalcoholic fatty liver disease (NAFLD). Fatty liver refers to the accumulation of fats in hepatocytes that usually occurs due to heavy drinking. When alcohol is not the cause, the sources are diabetes, hyperlipidemia, or a metabolic syndrome. The risk also increases due to such factors as a sedentary lifestyle; high cholesterol; underactivity of the endocrine system, particularly the thyroid and pituitary glands; and gastric bypass surgery. NAFLD can lead to a more severe form called nonalcoholic steatohepatitis (NASH).[6]

Unfortunately, there is evidence suggesting that genetic predisposition can influence the chance of developing hepatitis. Autoimmune hepatitis is induced when the immune system attacks liver cells that are otherwise undamaged. It is linked with the abnormal presence of certain human leukocyte antigens. Females have a much higher risk of developing this disease, particularly at a young age, as do people troubled by other autoimmune diseases. If there is family history of autoimmune hepatitis, it is important to still check for liver damage, even if there are no symptoms.[7]

VIRAL RISK FACTORS FOR HEPATITIS

By far the most common cause of hepatitis is a virus. There are five distinct hepatitis viruses: hepatitis A virus (HAV), hepatitis B virus (HBV), hepatitis C virus (HCV), hepatitis D virus (HDV), and hepatitis E virus (HEV).[8]

There is one antigen common to every HAV, a single-stranded RNA picornavirus. The virus is present in the fecal matter of an infected person and is spread via the fecal–oral route. This means that food or water is contaminated with particles of infected stool and then ingested by the victim. HAV can survive for months in water and is highly resistant to detergents, acids, and solvents. Temperatures of more than 140 degrees Fahrenheit are required to kill it. In developing countries, the risk of infection can reach close to 100 percent and is usually contracted during childhood. The virus is exterminated through treatments with medically formulized chlorine, formalin, peracetic acid, and UV radiation.[9]

Factors that increase the risk of infection include traveling to or living in highly endemic regions, working with children or in hospitals, and suffering from hemophilia or HIV. Living with an infected person is very risky. Rarely, certain unsafe sexual practices can proliferate the disease. The best method of prevention is vaccination.[10]

HBV is of the genus *Orthohepadnavirus*. In 1963, it was the first hepatitis virus to be identified. Similar viruses can be found in primates. Depending on the specific genotype of the virus, the disease it causes can be more or less severe. The genome consists of partially double-stranded DNA. It is an "enveloped" virus, and the particles of this envelope are required for hepatitis D infection. Hepatitis B is spread most commonly through blood, though other bodily fluids, such as semen, can carry it. Specific transmission methods are unprotected sex or contaminated equipment used for intravenous drugs, medical procedures, tattooing, and body piercing. Transfusions with infected blood are a major cause of disease. Even sharing such common items as razors and toothbrushes is potentially dangerous. Mother-to-child vertical transmission during childbirth contributes to the endemic nature of hepatitis B in areas like East Asia. Health-care workers, drug users, and those with multiple sexual partners are especially at risk of infection.[11]

HCV has a lipid envelope and contains a single strand of RNA. It belongs to the same family as the yellow fever virus, Flaviviridae. After infecting a hepatocyte in the liver, the virus causes it to generate about fifty virus particles, or virions, every day, with an average total of one trillion virions produced. There are seven genotypes of HCV, and the type that infects a person determines how antiviral drugs, such as interferon and ribavirin, are administered. HCV, like HBV, is emitted through blood. Unprotected sex or mother-to-child infections occur rarely. In developed countries, drug users are most susceptible to hepatitis C. Worldwide, post-transfusion infection is the most common. It is speculated that insect bites can also carry the disease from person to person.[12]

The hepatitis delta virus, or HDV, is a spherical RNA virus. A person can only develop hepatitis D when they also have HBV, so it is called a subviral satellite. Consequently, the overwhelming risk factor for HDV infection is previous HBV infection. It is transmitted through blood, and the people of the Mediterranean, sub-Saharan Africa, and northern South America have the highest rates of contamination. Worldwide, about 20 million people are infected with both viruses, potentially accelerating liver damage and the prospect of liver cancer.[13]

The genome of HEV is similar to that of the rubella virus. It is part of the Hepeviridae family and contains single-stranded RNA. It is transmitted through the fecal–oral route. Genotype 1 HEV is the most widespread. The majority of infections are caused by drinking contaminated water and eating raw shellfish collected from contaminated bodies of water. It is most prevalent in poorly developed areas with warm climates and where sewage disposal is an issue. HEV can also be present in domestic animals. Eating meat, particularly pork and derived products, originating from areas with high rates of infection presents a significant risk.[14]

ANALYSIS

The ultimate purpose of reviewing malicious microbes—of etiology, that is—is to develop methods to eliminate the prevalence of hepatitis at the global scale, as portrayed in chapter 7. The best method yet for reaching this goal is through extensive and systematic vaccination, as has been shown in such nations as the United States, where the rate of new viral hepatitis infection has plunged over the last few decades.[15]

10

DIAGNOSIS OF HEPATITIS

The clinical route for identifying disease based on signs and symptoms is referred to as diagnosis. For a person to reach an accurate diagnosis, a vast reserve of knowledge is essential. Diagnosis is a challenging occupation because many diseases share signs and symptoms with hepatitis, and there can be many symptomatic variations for any particular disease.[1]

The indisputable medical history of the hepatitis sufferer contributes to a doctor's decision making when considering a diagnosis. As knowledge of the relationships between signs and symptoms of various diseases accumulates, the process of diagnosis inevitably turns more accurate and specific. In some cases, a diagnosis may be pronounced even though the etiology, or cause, of the disorder cannot be identified. For example, the specific virus that causes hepatitis C was identified in the 1980s. However, the disease was known, diagnosed, and treated regularly prior to that time and was referred to as non-A, non-B hepatitis.[2]

The trigger for a diagnostic procedure is presumably the patient complaining of distress. Incidental discoveries can also serve as starting points, such as abnormal parameters of anatomy, homeostasis, or psychology during otherwise unrelated consultations. The diagnostician then records the symptoms expressed by the patient and observes visible signs. Some signs can be detected through physical inspection of areas of the body where the patient reports pain or disorder. The medical history of a patient is usually kept on file by one's personal or family doctor. Previous illness is a useful indication because the patient may be susceptible to relapse. In other cases, the patient develops immunity after a disease is eliminated, thus helping to eliminate some possible causes. Impaired functionality of certain organs or structures in the body helps pinpoint the exact location of an illness. It is also possible that the medical histories of the people that the patient comes in frequent contact with is useful. The sufferer's recent travel history, in conjunction with knowledge of epidemiology, can elucidate an unlikely source of infection.[3]

The process of diagnosis usually involves a combination of several methods. Pattern recognition is used by the expert during a consultation through the means described earlier. This may be sufficient for an illness that is common or seasonal and harmless in the long term, such as the common cold. Another method is differential diagnosis, which means that all the possible causes of a set of symptoms are considered, and through a subsequent process of elimination, the only possible cause or the smallest possible amount of causes, ordered by probability, remains. Clinical decision support systems are computer programs designed to help doctors reach accurate diagnosis. DXplain is one such program that has been used for more than twenty-five years, and IBM continues to improve an artificial intelligence software titled Watson.[4]

SCREENING FOR HEPATITIS

Screening is a medical procedure applied to large groups of people to catch a potential disease that has not yet manifested through widespread symptoms. Those who are screened are usually unaware of any specific health problems. Populations may be at risk of certain diseases due to epidemiological factors, and screening is used to (1) preempt the further distention of disease in a population, and (2) improve the treatment capacity of those afflicted. Screening tests must be specific when trying to identify a disease, such as hepatitis, because bias in scientific confirmations can have far-reaching costs.[5]

Hepatitis screening is done through blood tests. Serologic tests for the hepatitis B virus have been at the foundation of blood screening. Universal screening infers that everyone is tested regardless of the risk factors of each individual. Universal hepatitis screening is important in areas where the disease is prevalent. Blood donors are also universally tested worldwide. Otherwise, screening procedures are calibrated based on risk factors present in the population.[6]

Hepatitis B and C are transmitted through infected blood and are the most widespread forms of the disease, as well as the most deadly, with more than 400 million people infected worldwide and more than 1 million deaths annually. Depending on specific risk factors, individuals may be authorized for screening only once or periodically. Population groups approached for periodic screening include the following[7]:

- drug users, whether intravenous or intranasal;
- alcoholics;
- individuals incarcerated repeatedly;
- people who get tattoos or body piercings;
- those with frequent, high-risk sexual behavior; and
- health-care workers.

A single screening is normally recommended for persons whose parents have been infected with viral hepatitis and those born before widespread blood-screening procedures were implemented (1992 in the United States). The Centers for Disease Control and Prevention (CDC) recommends screening those born between 1945 and 1965. In developing countries, screening those who have undergone surgical procedures is key due to the frequency of intrahospital contamination.[8]

Hepatitis A screening is crucial in communities with poor sanitation levels and high frequency of water contamination. A single source of food or water can produce an outbreak very quickly. When a case of hepatitis A is reported in a small, tight-knit community, there is a high probability that screening the entire population will reveal high incidence levels of infection, in some cases reaching 100 percent.[9]

SEROLOGY IN THE SCHEME OF DIAGNOSIS

When physicians identify signs and symptoms in hepatitis patients, they request blood tests. The results of the blood tests are scrutinized, including the general chemistry, enzyme levels, and existence of antibodies. In some cases, physicians require an imaging analysis to identify lipid deposits in liver cells. A liver biopsy may be needed to hash out any cases of cirrhosis if previous tests do not successfully confirm its presence or lack thereof.[10]

In the case of viral hepatitis, it is diagnosed through antigen tests, nucleic acid tests, or serological tests. The hepatitis A virus is detected through a serological test. This is a blood screening for specific antibodies manufactured by the immune system in response to disease. If IgM anti-HAV antibodies are detected, then the patient is diagnosed with hepatitis A. However, if the patient has already had hepatitis A and purged it from the body, then IgG anti-HAV antibodies remain in the bloodstream and are detected by the test. These antibodies grant lifelong immunity from hepatitis A.[11]

Hepatitis B is diagnosed with the help of tests called assays that identify the antigens (proteins that are part of a virus) typical of the hepatitis B virus or antibodies produced after infection. The antigen HBsAg is the first to show up after infection, but after a period of time, it may be cleared by the patient. Thus, subsequent tests are performed to search for other antigens. These tests respond to different antigens, which also helps doctors determine the progress of disease. When a patient is determined to be infected with HBV, similar checks are done to investigate the possibility of coinfection with the hepatitis D virus.[12]

The serological test for hepatitis C provides results in less than thirty minutes. If it is inconclusive, a different method can be used. In nucleic acid tests (NATs), the virus can be witnessed more quickly than by simply seeking out antibodies. These tests search for the presence of genetic material (DNA or RNA) belonging to the virus. Tests are also used to determine the specific genotype of the virus, which determines the treatment applied to the patient. Acute hepatitis E is symptomatically indistinguishable from hepatitis A. With the exception of areas where hepatitis E is endemic, it is usually discovered through serological tests or NATs when the hepatitis A virus is eliminated as a cause.[13]

ANALYSIS

Careful and precise diagnostic procedures must be followed at all times. A wrong conclusion is called misdiagnosis, and it can have disastrous outcomes for a patient. Delayed diagnosis is equally dangerous because hepatitis may progress beyond the brackets of recovery.[14]

11

ROLE OF PRIMARY CARE PHYSICIANS

A person with an undiagnosed health issue will first contact a primary care physician. These experts have long-term relationships with their patients, providing comprehensive continuous medical care. A medical specialist is a professional with advanced training who sees patients after they have initially been to another physician and received a diagnosis. A hepatitis doctor is an example of one such specialist.[1]

TRAINING FOR PRIMARY CARE PROVIDERS

All who aspire to a medical career as a physician must attend an undergraduate school and receive a four-year bachelor of science (BS) or bachelor of arts (BA) degree from a university or college, generally with a great emphasis on basic sciences, such as biology, physics, or chemistry. Following that, a student must attend four years of medical school and obtain a degree. Finally, graduates branch off and undertake three to eight years in internship and residency programs (professional training under the supervision of senior mentor or attending physicians).[2]

Those who choose the primary care provider (PCP) path undergo a more generalized medical training program, consisting of three years of residency. This encompasses counseling and advising patients on good health habits, self-care, and options for treatment, as well as basic diagnosis, such as collecting information on the patient's medical background, current symptoms, and any other relevant health details. Next up are physical examinations, immunizations, and analysis of specific medical conditions, such as hepatitis and other common illnesses. Basic medical testing is also a requirement; examples include interpreting the results of a blood analysis, X-rays, and electrocardiograms.[3]

After a residency program of advanced education and clinical training in a specific domain of medicine, which usually takes more than three years, often comes a fellowship. This is a high specialization in a particular area of medicine that consists of between one and three years of additional training. Ranging from allergy and immunology to radiology and vascular surgery, specialists follow a very detailed training program related to their specific areas.[4]

A TYPICAL DAY FOR A PRIMARY CARE PHYSICIAN

A primary care physician's job is not easy, but it is essential. The time and energy needed extends health care beyond technical competence. In a typical day, a PCP begins by visiting and managing patients, sometimes in several hospitals, for up to three hours, followed by office hours, which can last from six to ten hours a day. They also usually receive a high number of phone calls from hospital doctors, who need to discuss the ongoing care of individuals with hepatitis, and patients or their family members to follow up or discuss health status.[5]

INITIAL APPOINTMENTS

The long-term relationship between a PCP and his patient should be a partnership in the interest of the patient's health. The PCP needs to review a person's previous medical records for any past conditions, illnesses, and treatments, including childhood diseases, chronic illnesses, and hospitalizations. The PCP also needs to know past and present prescriptions and over-the-counter medications that the patient is or has been taking. Also, it is important to let the doctor know of any allergies or adverse reactions to medications. Any additional data about the patient's psychological state and lifestyle relevant to health can be very useful for the PCP to procure an accurate picture of that person's life. When it comes to hepatitis, the PCP should recognize the symptoms that go with each type of the disease.[6]

For HAV, the most common symptom is fading energy. Additionally, loss of appetite, headaches, itchy skin, muscle soreness, and pain near the liver can occur. Sometimes the patient may also experience jaundice. The incubation of this strand of hepatitis ranges from fifteen to fifty days. Within seven to eight weeks, the symptoms often go away. HAV itself usually exits after about a half-year. The primary physician should order a blood test to detect HAV antibodies in the body. If the test is positive, then bedrest is recommended, along with avoiding alcohol, consuming a lot of fluids, and eating a healthy diet. The best way to prevent HAV is the hepatitis A vaccination.[7]

HBV symptoms include loss of appetite, nausea, fever, tiredness, headaches, sore muscles, pain near the liver, and jaundice. However, many with HBV have no symptoms at all. The incubation period ranges from 30 to 150 days, with an average of 90 days. As with HAV, diagnostic blood tests are done to see if HBV antibodies are present. In the case of acute HBV, there is no need for medication. Chronic HBV, however, cannot be cured, and the patient might enter and remain in an inactive hepatitis B surface antigen (HBsAg) carrier phase. PCPs should immunize everyone, from infants to adolescents as well as adults at risk of contracting HBV. In addition to clinical and laboratory evaluation, screening should be done for folks at high risk. If a patient is identified as HBsAg positive, then they need to be monitored, and the PCP will often consult with a specialist.[8]

As with hepatitis B, most people infected with HCV do not experience symptoms. However, they do have mild, flulike symptoms, such as tiredness, sore muscles, joint pain, fever, nausea, poor appetite, stomach pain, itchy skin, dark urine, and jaundice. The incubation period of HCV ranges from 15 to 160 days, with an average of 50 days. Primary care physicians should screen all patients at risk of HCV. After identifying a risk factor, an initial test for HCV, which uses an enzyme-linked immunoassay (ELIZA) to identify antibodies for HCV, is done. Detection of these antibodies can be done within four to ten weeks after infection, but they cannot distinguish between a previous or a new chronic infection. Another test, an HCV RNA assay that can be qualitative or quantitative, can be done to assert the presence of the virus. The PCP should identify risk factors for the patient that may lead to discovering the original time of infection. Counseling the patient about preventing HCV transmission is also very important. A comprehensive laboratory profile conducted by the physician is very helpful for treatment specialists and allows them to propose a more comprehensive consultation with the first patient visit. Although the nonphysician caregivers cannot medically treat the patient, it is always a good idea for everyone to educated themselves about the disease, drug treatment, side effects, and dangers of overdose.[9]

ANALYSIS

From a patient's perspective, preparing for the first appointment with a PCP builds the foundation for a good doctor–patient relationship, which is important for better care and continuing good health. The PCP needs to understand the strategies for treating hepatitis and its multiple side effects and help the patient complete the full course of treatment. Helping the patient to believe in the treatment is equally vital.[10]

12

ROLE OF HEPATOLOGISTS

Hepatologists are medical professionals who have the most experience and training in dealing with diseases of the liver. Their care is usually sought when other physicians do not have the required experience or qualifications to correctly diagnose and treat patients suffering from liver illnesses.[1]

TRAINING FOR HEPATOLOGISTS

After completing their undergraduate degrees and four years of medical school, much like students looking to become primary care providers, aspiring hepatologists complete a three-year residency, where the student comes in contact with a variety of clinical and research opportunities relating to diagnosis and treatment of diseases affecting nearly all organs. In contrast to primary caregivers, hepatology students continue their studies by attending a fellowship program in gastroenterology and hepatology for an additional three years. This is where the skills and training for treating patients with liver, pancreas, and gallbladder diseases are refined.[2]

INITIAL APPOINTMENTS

When preparing for an appointment with a hepatologist, the patient should be well prepared. Patients should know of any preappointment tasks, such as dietary restrictions. Furthermore, taking notes during the appointment or taking a family member or friend along can be helpful to keep track of all the information received. Before attending the first appointment, the patient can compile a list of questions about the extent of their infection; the damage it may have caused to the liver; treatment options, with their risks and benefits; foods, drinks, and medications to avoid; and the dangers of spreading the disease to others. The hepatologist will probably ask questions about symptoms, such as when they first started and if anything improves or worsens them. Among other things, a patient can expect to be asked if their family has a history of the disease, if they ever had blood transfusions or a transplant, and if they have ever used self-injected drugs.[3]

A hepatologist will perform a number of medical tests and analyses, ranging from physical examinations and blood analysis to endoscopies, liver biopsies, and bilirubin analysis. They can also prescribe medication and recommend genetic screening and liver transplants.[4]

Each strand of viral hepatitis is different in progression and danger level, and not all types of infection requires the care of a hepatologist. HAV is eliminated in the stool toward the end of its incubation period, so treatments are adjusted to best fit the patient's age, medical history, and stage of infection, with the goal of reducing liver damage and treating any complications that may arise. HAV antibodies are discerned between one to two weeks after initial infection and remain visible for three to four months. Their presence signifies the end of the acute stage, and the patient will be immune to further infection. In this case, consulting a hepatologist is not necessary, as long as the diagnosis is correct.[5]

The case is similar with acute HBV, with most patients experiencing symptoms in the early stages of infection. The illness itself actually lasts for a few weeks, and the patient gradually improves. However, there are a few incidents where a complication may occur and result in acute liver failure. Chronic HBV is more dangerous because of its long-term nature and the potential for cirrhosis and liver cancer. If diagnosed with chronic HBV, consultation with an experienced liver specialist, gastroenterologist, or hepatologist is a must. Frequent visits to the specialist are not required, unless undergoing treatment; in some cases, more blood work and monitoring are warranted, but this is usually for short periods of time. Therapy is necessary for patients with a high level of HBV replication and active or advanced liver disease in order to lower HBV DNA levels, stabilize serum alanine aminotransferase, and improve liver histology. This can vary from six months to a year. Even though there are no available medications that can clear the infection, there are medications that can stop the replication of the virus, thus minimizing liver damage.[6]

Another danger imposed by HBV is coinfection, or superimposed infection, with HDV, which only occurs in association with HBV. The presence of this satellite strand of hepatitis can further endanger the patient and lead to liver failure and other severe complications. Hepatologists will recommend avoiding alcohol as well as any medications that might worsen hepatic function. For acute infections, supportive care is recommended, whereas for chronic cases, interferon is needed. The reactivation of HBV is possible, as the virus persists in the body, although it is rare. People who undergo immunity-impairing treatments, such as chemotherapy, are at high risk, as are drug users. Alcohol can also reactivate the virus.[7]

HCV is the most dangerous strand and accounts for the most liver transplants. A person at risk of HCV should first consult a family doctor or general practitioner; if they are diagnosed with HCV, then they must see a specialist. It is recommended that testing is done as early as possible for high-risk patients because the disease can potentially do grave damage to the liver before any signs or symptoms appear. It is imperative to consider lifestyle changes (at the doctor's recommendation) and begin treatment as soon as possible to prevent this from happening.[8]

The hepatologist will order blood tests to measure the viral load (quantity of HCV) and evaluate the genetic makeup of the virus, which determines the patient's treatment options. A biopsy will most likely be required, as it is the most accurate way to evaluate the severity of liver damage. This is done by inserting a needle through the patient's skin and into the liver to collect a tissue sample. This poses a small risk of complication, most commonly bleeding, but other risks include bile leak, intestinal perforation, and full-blown hemophilia. The latter examplcs arc extremely rare. Therapy usually ceases after twelve months, especially if no response has been observed. Patients who develop cirrhosis or liver cancer may need to undergo a liver transplant.[9]

A laboratory location that fulfills the sensitivity requirements for hepatitis testing and is close to the patient should be found. HCV patients also need counseling about pregnancy during their therapy and for six months following their last treatment. HCV therapy is difficult, with side effects including mood swings and depression. The hepatologist must communicate and encourage their patients while undergoing therapy.[10]

ANALYSIS

Hepatologists monitor patients, some who live at great distances from the clinic or hospital. For the most successful care, patients should keep a log of symptoms, medications (including vitamins and supplements), and recent significant life changes that have had an impact on stress levels.[11]

13

ROLE OF GASTROENTEROLOGISTS

A gastroenterologist is a physician with dedicated training and unique experience in the care of the gastrointestinal (GI) tract and liver, including the esophagus, pancreas, intestines, and colon, as well as their accessory glands. Acid reflux, irritable bowel syndrome, and Crohn's disease are just a small batch of illnesses they are certified to diagnose. Gastroenterologists can also perform endoscopies, which help identify or in some cases remove diseased portions of the digestive tract. They also work closely with primary care physicians and surgeons.[1]

TRAINING FOR GASTROENTEROLOGISTS

Training to become a gastroenterologist takes years of medical study. From undergraduate studies through medical school, specialized residency, and fellowship training in gastroenterology, students have in total around ten years of medical training. Their path is similar to that of hepatologists. Hepatologists are considered subspecialists of gastroenterology, but differences in specialized training exist.[2]

During fellowship, a gastroenterologist in training undergoes an intense and rigorous program where they learn how to evaluate patients with GI complaints and give out recommendations and treatment to maintain or improve health. These doctors receive dedicated guidance in endoscopy, including detailed studies on how and when to optimally and safely perform such tests. They also learn advanced endoscopic techniques, such as biliary examinations, removal of colon polyps, or even removal of tumors without surgery. Because the liver is part of the digestive system, gastroenterologists are trained in treating many forms of liver-related disorders, including hepatitis.[3]

However, a gastroenterologist's level of expertise in diagnosing and treating liver disease may vary greatly. During the course of their residency, some gastroenterologists may have very little exposure to patients with liver disease, whereas others might have a great deal. Hepatologists' training, on the other hand, is focused solely on liver-related illnesses, making them the most experienced and qualified doctors to treat individuals with liver ailments.[4]

Even though gastroenterologists who have not completed a fellowship in hepatology may devote their medical practice primarily to the diagnosis and treatment of people with liver disease, a person should choose to see a hepatologist. If a hepatologist is not available in an area and there is convenient access to a gastroenterologist instead, then the patient should determine the doctor's level of expertise in liver disease before instituting a perpetual doctor–patient relationship.[5]

Many people are diagnosed with hepatitis by their primary care provider. Depending on the strand of this disease, PCPs may be able to offer treatment to patients suffering from hepatitis, though in the more serious cases with risk of complications, a specialist needs to be consulted. In these situations, the best option is a gastroenterologist or hepatologist.[6]

A TYPICAL DAY FOR GASTROENTEROLOGISTS

Usually, gastroenterologists spend half the week at the office and the other half at the hospitals in which they work. An average office day starts off with about eight or nine procedures from morning to afternoon, followed by patient visits in the office. Typical hospital days have the doctor performing five to seven endoscopies. They also see several patients on their rounds and offer around five new consultations per day. The workload is high, and they must also keep up with new developments and research.[7]

INITIAL APPOINTMENTS

Initial appointments with a gastroenterologist are much like appointments with a regular physician. They will ask for the patient's medical history and symptoms, after which they may perform a physical examination. Following this, the doctor and patient will discuss the need for additional tests, therapy options, and medications. The gastroenterologist will recommend an endoscopy or colonoscopy and an abdominal ultrasound, which will be scheduled for later visits.[8]

Before the first appointment, patients should ask the doctor if there is anything in particular they need to bring or if they should perform any specific tasks. The patient's primary care physician should forward the reason of referral, in addition to copies of laboratory results, blood work, X-ray reports, and so on, to the gastroenterologist. It is also best if the patient brings a list of symptoms, medications, allergies, and past illnesses to the first appointment. Notetaking during the visit is also helpful, as the amount of information received can be too much to remember. The patient should also verify if their insurance covers a gastroenterologist or if they need prior authorization, such as a referral from the PCP. It is best to check with the insurance company and get all the necessary details before scheduling an appointment.[9]

Blood tests tell the doctor what he needs to know, but a liver biopsy may also be required. With HBV and HCV, screening blood tests might be done to identify the infection because symptoms could show up only after the liver has already been damaged. HAV and acute HBV generally do not require medication, except perhaps for remedying symptoms. The body can fight the infection on its own, so rest and hydration are recommended. When HBV becomes chronic or for HCV, it may take monitoring and strong antiviral drugs to suppress complications. In both scenarios, the danger of serious liver damage and liver failure is looming and can lead to a liver transplant.[10]

ANALYSIS

Gastroenterology has high rewards, as this occupation also plays an incalculable part in the effort to reduce the death rate of one of America's biggest cancers. They are making great progress in screening people for colon cancer. Their methods can also help spare patients from major operations.[11]

14

ROLE OF HOSPITALS

Hospitals are health-care facilities with specialized medical staff and equipment, providing a patient with medical and surgical treatment. There are multiple types of hospitals: general, district, and specialized. A general hospital is set up to deal with a large variety of illnesses and injuries, including an emergency department prepared to deal with the most urgent and immediate health threats. District hospitals are major health-care institutions in a region that provide intensive care. Specialized hospitals include a number of dedicated medical facilities, such as teaching hospitals, children's hospitals, geriatric hospitals, psychiatric and rehabilitation hospitals, and trauma centers.[1]

A hospital is divided into working departments. Urgent care, surgery, intensive care, and cardiology are just a few departments that a hospital may have. They can also include support units, such as radiology or a pharmacy. Certain hospitals have chronic treatment units for diseases such as hepatitis. Generally, people with hepatitis don't need to be admitted to a hospital. They can undergo their necessary treatments or diagnostic tests as outpatients, treated by a primary care physician, hepatologist, or gastroenterologist. In case of a chronic infection, depending on the stage of the disease, patients may need to be hospitalized, especially if the virus has already damaged the liver.[2]

Hospitals offer a sterile environment, especially when dealing with patients who have contagious and infectious diseases, like hepatitis. With a risk of exposure to a contagious disease, caregivers working in such environments should receive corresponding vaccinations while monitoring and testing their immunity. Hepatitis A and E, for instance, may be transmitted through fecal–oral exchanges in hospitals. A patient infected with these types of hepatitis can infect a healthy person through direct contact in a hospital or indirectly through food and water if they failed to wash their hands properly after using the restroom. Hepatitis B, C, and D are spread through exposure to infected blood and other bodily fluids. Hospital-based caregivers should adhere to fundamental infection-control principles and standard precautions to prevent transmission of blood-borne pathogens. These include proper aseptic practices and safe injection techniques. Reusing needles and syringes can result in direct transmission of the virus to other patients or infection of hemodialysis units.[3]

Hygiene is the mechanism for disease prevention in any sickbay, including cleaning and disinfecting the patient's surroundings, laundry, and bedding. In some cases, for patients suffering from other contagious diseases, extra precautions need to be taken. For example, a patient with an airborne infectious disease must be treated in an isolated room with special ventilation systems.[4]

INPATIENT AND OUTPATIENT SETTINGS

Not all patients at a hospital are inpatients, who need overnight or a longer admission. Patients who go to a hospital for a diagnosis or therapy and then leave are called outpatients. Outpatient care can be afforded in a clinic, doctor's office, or even a patient's home. Advances in treatment and technology have made procedures that were formerly only conducted in a hospital possible in an office setting. Outpatient care can include treatment for chemical dependency, mental health problems, and chronic diseases. Physical therapy and chemotherapy are also involved. In these cases, the benefits of choosing a hospital over a clinic include more specialized equipment and expertise. An inpatient can discuss their treatment options and help plan their care while always having the right to refuse treatment. They will then sign an informed consent explaining the tests, treatments, and procedures, or they can have someone else sign it for them if they are unable to do so themselves.[5]

While admitted into a hospital for hepatitis, a patient's activity is limited to reduce abdominal injury. Caregivers will gather information about the patient's current state by checking temperature, blood pressure, heart rate, and breathing rate. During their stay at the hospital, inpatients have a special diet and avoid alcohol. Patients are hooked up to an intravenous (IV) system, which provides medicine through a small tube inserted into a vein. Blood samples are taken either directly from the patient or from the IV to monitor enzymes and other substances given off by the liver. Other tests can include a liver biopsy to check for swelling, scarring, or any other damage and an abdominal ultrasound, which can also help identify liver problems. For hepatitis C patients, there are additional blood tests required. An enzyme immunoassay test checks for HCV antibodies present in the blood, while a hepatitis C profile serological test focuses on the number of viruses in the blood and checks activity. Genotyping, another blood test, informs the doctors on how long the patient needs treatment by identifying the genotype of the present HCV virus.[6]

Hepatitis therapy for inpatients consists of antiviral medicine to decelerate the multiplication of the virus. These can include adefovir, lamivudine, tenofovir, telbivudine, and such immune system modulators as interferons with ribavirin. Hepatitis B immunoglobulin is given to patients and newborns exposed to the virus in the womb. If the patient has problems with their blood not clotting properly, then they will receive a plasma or platelet transfusion trough an IV. Surgery might be needed to remove a part of the liver or even a liver transplant is needed for life-threatening conditions. In this situation, specialists from varying fields need to determine if a transplant is appropriate and choose donor candidates. If the new liver is not a good match, then the body may reject it.[7]

Every treatment is a gamble. Hepatitis B may cause liver damage even with treatment, whereas without it, there is the chance of HVB becoming chronic (increasing the possibility of liver scarring and failure) or developing an abdominal infection leading to bleeding in the stomach and esophagus. Patients undergoing cancer treatment or consuming certain medications, such as those for HIV, autoimmune disorders, and organ or bone marrow transplants, have more risks. Hepatitis C treatment poses a new set of ailments, such as headaches, depression, or even kidney damage. The earlier HCV is detected and treated, the better the chances of preventing further complications.[8]

OUTCOME OF TREATMENT

Health-care-related exposures are an uncommon source of viral hepatitis transmission in the United States, but there have been a few reported cases of HBV and HCV outbreaks in these settings. These incidents generally have the same cause: transmission from patient to patient through exposure to contaminated injection equipment with blood from one or more patients with a hepatitis virus. To prevent such incidents, training programs have reinforced infection-control principles and practices for those who work in outpatient settings.[9]

ANALYSIS

One of the most important factors in quality care for hepatitis is the collaboration between primary care physicians and specialists in hospitals. Larger care-management organizations, such as hospitals, offer the best equipment and specialists for diagnosing and treating both outpatients and inpatients with a hepatitis infection. They have an adequate environment for inpatients, as well as caring and competent staff, but it is important to ensure that PCPs remain informed of procedures done on patients.[10]

III

Many Faces of Hepatitis

15

HEPATITIS AND CHOLESTEROL

Cholesterol is a lipid molecule biosynthesized by internal organs; it is an essential substance for the normal functioning cells in the body. Cholesterol maintains the structural integrity, fluidity, and membranes of cells. It is oil based, unlike blood, which is water based, so it is carried throughout the body by lipoproteins in the blood. Cholesterol can also be ingested through certain foods.[1]

In addition to its importance for cells, cholesterol is a key factor in the structural makeup of certain hormones and digestive bile acids, and it enables the production of vitamin D in the body. Hepatitis authorities confirm that the balance of cholesterol is not only beneficial to the heart but also to the brain and liver, as it reduces brain plaque, which is linked to Alzheimer's disease.[2]

MAINTAINING PROPER CHOLESTEROL

A satisfactory balance of cholesterol consists of boosted levels of high-density lipoprotein (HDL), also known as good cholesterol, and lower levels of bad cholesterol, low-density lipoprotein (LDL). One of the major perils of high cholesterol levels, also known as hypercholesterolemia or hyperlipidemia, is coronary heart disease, which can cause heart attacks. Aberrantly low cholesterol levels, also called hypolipoproteinemia or hypolipidemia, can occur through malnutrition, hyperthyroidism, cancer, genetic disease, and liver disease.[3]

Raised cholesterol can be a result of a number of things, including diet, weight, activity level, age, and gender. A number of drugs and diseases, such as diabetes, chronic kidney disease, liver disease, or hypothyroidism, can also elevate cholesterol concentrations in a patient's bloodstream. However, the primary source of hyperlipidemia seems to be genetic. Conditions such as familial hyperlipidemia, familial hypertriglyceridemia, and dysbetalipoproteinemia can be inherited from parents.[4]

High cholesterol is only diagnosed through blood tests. To obtain an accurate reading, patients must abstain from drinks (except water), food, and pills for nine to twelve hours before screening. These blood tests provide information on total cholesterol levels, low-density and high-density lipoprotein levels, and triglyceride levels. Desired levels for total cholesterol are less than 200 milligrams per deciliter; optimal LDL levels are under 100 milligrams per deciliter. Hepatitis specialists recommend that people above the age of twenty review their levels at least once every five years.[5]

Not smoking and eating a low-fat diet can help manage these levels. It is best to avoid animal products, such as meat, eggs, and cheese, as well as deep-fried and processed foods containing saturated fats. Exercise also helps regulate cholesterol because being overweight or obese contributes to higher levels of low-density lipoproteins.[6]

For those with an impending risk of heart attack, diet and exercise may not be enough. In these cases, lipid-lowering drugs, known as statins, are available. Statins are also called HMG CoA reductase inhibitors and include pravastatin, atorvastatin, fluvastatin, lovastatin, and simvastatin. Depending on the overall heart risk, medication is recommended for people with cholesterol levels between 130 and 190 milligrams per deciliter. Other drugs that are used include cholesterol-absorption inhibitors, resins, niacin, and fibrates. Statins come with their share of side effects, such as low energy during exercise and fatigue. Researchers have also linked statin drugs to cataracts, but side effects are not typical, and practitioners say the benefits outweigh the risks.[7]

HEPATITIS AND CHOLESTEROL

Studies have shown that people with hepatitis C were more likely to have hypolipidemia—a lower level of total plasma cholesterol, low-density lipoproteins, and triglycerides—and a lower incidence of hyperlipidemia than the uninfected. Hypolipidemia in a patient infected by hepatitis C resolves itself with successful HCV treatment but is persistent in some patients, known as nonresponders. There is a potential danger for patients with successful HCV therapy: Cholesterol levels can rebound to levels that increase the risk of coronary artery disease (CAD), the most widespread type of heart disease, attributed to the buildup of plaque along the inner walls of the heart's arteries. The result is a near-stagnation of blood flow to the heart, which can lead to heart attacks. This is why monitoring lipid levels in patients undergoing hepatitis therapy is crucial.[8]

Prolonged infection with hepatitis B contributes to the inverse relationship between liver cancer and cholesterol concentration. A liver with extended hepatitis B infection, starting from childhood and persisting throughout adulthood, lowers the concentration of cholesterol in the blood of adults over time. This could help explain the significant inverse association between cholesterol levels and mortality rate from liver cancer and other chronic liver diseases.[9]

There is evidence of correlation between higher levels of bad cholesterol and a sustained virologic response to hepatitis C treatment. A strong virologic response means the virus has not been detected in the patient's blood six months after therapy has concluded and is considered a cure by many physicians. Research has associated high concentrations of low-density lipoprotein cholesterol with a better response to HCV treatment in people with both HCV and HIV infections. This is interesting, indeed, because one of the more problematic side effects of antiretroviral drugs is an increase in bad cholesterol levels and, thus, could actually be advantageous for people getting care for hepatitis C. A high level of low-density lipoprotein cholesterol has become an independent predictor of sustained virologic response to pegylated interferon with ribavirin (the most common medication used for HCV patients) in HCV and coinfected HCV/HIV patients alike.[10]

ANALYSIS

Test tube studies have found a cooperative interaction between certain drugs to lower cholesterol (especially fluvastatin) and hepatitis C treatment. It seems that these statin drugs amplify the effects of alpha interferon, resulting in a much more effective treatment than the common combination of interferon with ribavirin. With regards to fluvastatin, however, the effective concentration is roughly ten times higher than the normal concentration found in the blood of patients taking daily doses of the drug. Another conundrum is the fact that statin drugs can damage the liver. Further research and development could yield more effective drugs in the fight against hepatitis C.[11]

16

HEPATITIS AND OBESITY

Body fat is necessary for insulation, energy, and other functions. Obesity is a medical condition defined by an excess amount of body fat. It can cause all sorts of negative effects on the body, such as liver problems and a shorter life expectancy. The body mass index (BMI) is normally used to define obesity. The BMI is the ratio of a person's weight in kilograms to the squared value of their height in meters. In an adult, a BMI between 25 and 29.9 falls into the overweight category, while values over 30 indicate obesity.[1]

THE OBESITY SITUATION

Obesity has seen a rapid increase throughout the world in the last decades, with numbers doubling between 1991 and 1998. In the United States, obesity has become a severe problem, with two-thirds of adults being overweight. In America, obesity is the cause for approximately 112,000 deaths per year, with most of the victims having a BMI higher than 30. For those who have a BMI over 40, life expectancy is significantly reduced. Obesity can increase the prospect of a number of diseases, most of which are heart related. Apart from hypertension, high cholesterol, heart attacks, and strokes, obesity can also contribute to insulin resistance, type 2 diabetes, osteoarthritis, and even the pathological expansion of a number of cancers. In the case of high blood pressure, the distribution of fat in the body plays a role in the stages of disease. People with central obesity, also known as abdominal obesity, are at a higher risk of having high blood pressure than people who have fat mainly along the thighs and hips.[2]

Cholesterol concentration and high blood pressure have already been linked with hepatitis to a certain degree. The fact that obesity directly contributes to these conditions enforces the need for hepatitis patients to maintain their weight at healthy levels or to manage and reduce weight in cases of obesity. Even though the main cause of obesity is physical inactivity and overeating, there are a number of other contributing factors, such as genetics, metabolism, and medications.[3]

Overeating, especially with a diet rich in fats and sugar, will lead to weight gain. Fried foods, fast foods, and sweets tend to have a high energy density, meaning a high number of calories in a small amount of food. Carbohydrates may also play a role in weight gain. They activate glucose production in the blood, which in turn can stimulate the discharge of insulin by the pancreas. This may cause weight gain by encouraging the growth of fat tissue.[4]

Slow metabolism, which is another contributing factor to obesity, is a result of a reduction in muscle mass. Muscle burns more calories than any other tissue. This makes women more predisposed to a slower metabolism than men, who have comparatively more muscle mass. With aging, muscle mass tends to decrease, thus encouraging weight gain, especially if the person's daily caloric intake is not reduced.[5]

Several types of drugs are also associated with weight gain. Some of these include certain anticonvulsants, antidepressants, diabetes medication, and hormone drugs such as oral contraceptives and corticosteroids. Antihistamines and high blood pressure medication has also been noted to encourage weight gain. Reasons for this differ with each drug and should be discussed with a doctor.[6]

Adding to the obesity epidemic are a number of conditions, such as Cushing's syndrome, hypothyroidism, and insulin resistance. Finally, there is also a psychological dynamic to weight gain. Anger, stress, and sadness can influence some people's eating habits.[7]

MAINTAINING WEIGHT

Dealing with obesity is a struggle for many hepatitis sufferers. In many cases, lost weight can quickly return, even after strenuous dieting. People undertaking therapy must acknowledge that treatment takes a long time, but even modest weight loss and maintenance can have significant impact, such as lowering blood pressure, reducing cholesterol, and decreasing the risk of a stroke and heart disease. Exercise and physical activity can help scorch calories. However, exercise alone without changes to diet will have a very limited effect because losing even a single pound just by exercise takes a lot of work.[8]

With dieting, the first goal is to stop additional weight gain, followed by establishing realistic weight-loss goals. Reducing calorie intake per day for an obese hepatitis sufferer will have relatively quick results; more calories are required to maintain more weight. Long-term diets need to be planned carefully to be safe and effective. Diets have to be balanced and contain lower-energy-density, nutritious foods in order to avoid vitamin deficiency and malnutrition.[9]

Individuals with a BMI greater than 30 who are at risk of heart disease can use medication to help them control their weight. Medication should only be used in conjunction with an exercise and diet program. A certain group of drugs used to fight obesity, such as phentermine and sibutramine, create a sensation of fullness and also decrease appetite. The major side effect of these remedies is high blood pressure. Another class of drugs, called lipase inhibitors, prevents the metabolism of fat in the intestines by constraining digestive enzymes called lipases. Side effects of these drugs include changes in bowel movement.[10]

THE LIVER, HEPATITIS, AND OBESITY

In people with a chronic hepatitis C infection, obesity can influence insulin resistance, trigger inflammation, add to the progression of fibrosis, and even inhibit the response to treatment with interferon and ribavirin. This increases the risk of advanced liver disease in hepatitis patients. How obesity interferes with a sustained virologic response (SVR) to hepatitis C treatment is unclear, but theories do exist, one of which is that the abnormal immune response to therapy is due to the inflammatory condition of obesity. Another theory is that obesity can cause hepatic steatosis and insulin resistance, which may lead to liver fibrosis and steatohepatitis, thereby causing an interference with interferon therapy. Some speculate that patients with high levels of subcutaneous fat may not be able to properly absorb pegylated interferon alpha administered via subcutaneous injections. If the volume of the drug absorbed by the body is less than the dose required, then the treatment could be unsuccessful.[11]

ANALYSIS

Hepatitis C patients with obesity should first be encouraged to exercise and lose weight. This will reduce fibrosis and steatosis, in addition to reducing serum triglyceride concentration and blood pressure. Treating insulin resistance before or together with antiviral therapy might also lead to improvements in hepatitis C patients. Other ways to improve the response to pegylated interferon and ribavirin treatment in overweight patients are higher doses of the drugs or longer duration of therapy. These strategies, dedicated to improving underlying metabolic conditions, should increase the rate of the physiological response in individuals with hepatitis.[12]

17

HEPATITIS AND HEART DISEASE

Heart and blood vessel disease, also called cardiovascular disease, refers to all disorders related to the cardiovascular system. Cardiovascular disease is the number one cause of fatality in the United States. Hepatitis C patients should pay extra attention to their cardiovascular health because HCV is a risk factor for coronary artery disease.[1]

CARDIOVASCULAR CONDITIONS

There are a number of conditions that can cause these illnesses, but the most common are hypertension and atherosclerosis. The latter is caused by buildup of a substance called plaque on the blood vessel's inner walls. The result of this buildup is the narrowing of the arteries, which makes blood flow a lot harder and increases the risk of blood clots. Blood clots can completely cut blood flow to parts of the heart, causing the muscles in that area to decay. A blood clot severely increases the risk of a heart attack. The majority of people will survive their first heart attack, but depending on the degree of heart disease and damage that was caused, doctors will recommend some serious changes in lifestyle and medication.[2]

Blood clotting can also trigger strokes when the channels of the blood vessels supplying the brain are congested. Similar to a heart attack, a lack of blood circulation to any part of the brain will cause the decay of cells and shut down of the brain in the affected region. This can render a person incapable of carrying out normal functions, such as walking or talking. Some brain cells may only be injured and can heal themselves over time, but with cells that die due to lack of oxygen and blood, the damage is permanent. This type of stroke is called an ischemic stroke and represents the vast majority of stroke cases. Unrestrained hypertension is the cause for another type of stroke called hemorrhagic stroke, which causes blood vessels inside the brain to burst.[3]

Heart failure, also called congestive or chronic heart failure, is when the heart is incapable of pumping the blood required to supply the body. This condition can quickly deteriorate if not handled in time. Heart failure is most commonly caused by coronary artery disease, high blood pressure, and cardiomyopathy.[4]

Other cardiovascular diseases include arrhythmia and heart valve problems. Arrhythmia refers to abnormal rhythms of the heart. A low heart rate, with fewer than sixty beats per minute, is known as bradycardia, whereas a high heart rate with more than one hundred beats per minute is called tachycardia. Arrhythmia can cause a problem similar to heart failure by shifting the normal function of the heart and not supplying the body with the blood it needs. Valvular problems refer to either blood leaks due to the heart's valves not closing properly (regurgitation) or low blood flow due to incorrect valve opening (stenosis).[5]

CARDIOVASCULAR DISEASE SIGNS AND SYMPTOMS

Each type of heart disease has its own treatment, but most share similar warning signs. Coronary artery disease often causes palpitations, weakness, pain in the chest (angina), shortness of breath, and dizziness. A heart attack can start with mild chest discomfort that then radiates to the back, arm, throat, or jaw and eventually proceeds to significant pain. Other heart attack symptoms include extreme weakness, dizziness, irregular heartbeats, and a choking sensation. Heart attack symptoms generally last for thirty minutes or more, and it is imperative to call for emergency help immediately.[6]

For heart failure, heart valve disease, and arrhythmia, symptoms do not necessarily relate to the severity of the condition. These illnesses share the symptoms of chest discomfort, shortness of breath, weakness, dizziness, and palpitations. In addition to these, heart failure can result in coughs that render white sputum; rapid weight gain; and swelling in the legs, ankles, or abdomen. Other signs may include fainting and pounding in the chest.[7]

DIAGNOSING CARDIOVASCULAR DISEASE

Cardiovascular disease is diagnosed with simple techniques and tests, such as a physical examination, heart rate, heartbeat, blood pressure, and blood tests. Later, more advanced assessments can be done.[8]

Electrocardiograms (ECG or EKG) record the electrical activity of an individual's heart through small electrode patches attached to the arms, legs, and chest. Chest X-rays can also be performed to reveal signs of cardiac disease. Another procedure is an exercise stress test, also called an exercise ECG or stress ECG. This helps determine abnormal heart rhythms in patients and if blood flow to the heart is adequate during increased activity. Stress tests also help check the effectiveness of medication and procedures for hepatitis patients with coronary artery disease.[9]

Echocardiograms use sound waves to create moving pictures of the heart. These procedures evaluate the size and shape of the heart muscles as well as the functioning of the heart valves and chambers. Other tests to diagnose cardiac health are cardiac catheterization, tilt table tests, heart MRIs, heart CT scans, myocardial biopsies, and electrophysiology assessments.[10]

CARDIOVASCULAR DISEASE PREVENTION

Hepatitis sufferers should note the best ways to prevent cardiovascular disease are increasing physical activity and exercise per day; eating high-fiber, low-fat diets that include fruits, vegetables, and whole grains; and reducing sugar intake. Quitting or avoiding smoking and limiting alcohol consumption can decrease the risk of heart disease by 30 percent. For overweight or obese people, maintaining good blood pressure levels and decreasing body fat will also dramatically reduce the risk of heart disease. Lastly, severe physical and emotional stress is known to lead to heart problems. Thus, dropping the stress levels can help prevent heart malfunctions.[11]

The customary ways of lessening the risk of heart disease might not be enough for people with a hepatitis C infection. Besides the damage it can do to the liver, the hepatitis C virus can also harm the heart. Although a healthy lipid profile and blood pressure is fundamental for a healthy cardiovascular system, hepatitis C patients should take added steps. Because specialists believe that events that cause the virus to flare up also increase heart disease, all attempts need to be made to minimize the viral load of HCV. Additional treatment can include abstinence from alcohol, antioxidants (like alpha R-lipoic acid or NAC) to keep cells healthy, and milk thistle supplements to combat viral replication in the liver. Nattokinase supplements can also be useful, as they help to dissolve dangerous blood clots.[12]

ANALYSIS

An ultradistinct connection between hepatitis C and heart disease is yet to be unearthed. While numerous studies have shown that, on average, hepatitis C patients have lower blood pressure, decreased plasma and LDL cholesterol levels, and a reduced number of triglycerides compared to patients without hepatitis C, individuals with the virus seem to be at a higher risk of heart disease. Experts suggest that increased inflammation, immune activation, and blood clotting might be the culprits behind such an elevated cardiovascular risk.[13]

18

HEPATITIS AND LIVER CANCER

Cancer, also called tumors, is a class of deadly diseases involving abnormal cell growth that has the potential to proliferate to other parts of the body. There are more than one hundred distinctive cancers known to affect humans; each form is typified by the cell it initially targets. Hepatic cancer makes cells in the liver divide uncontrollably and form masses of tissue or lumps, referred to as tumors. These tumors release hormones that alter body function. As they grow and spread, they can also interfere with the circulatory, digestive, and nervous systems.[1]

Tumors that exhibit limited growth or no growth at all are called benign. Dangerous, malignant tumors can form when cancerous cells start to divide and grow, creating new blood vessels to feed themselves. This process is called angiogenesis. Hepatocytic tumors assault the liver. Metastasis is when the tumor successfully spreads to other parts of the body through the lymphatic or cardiovascular system, destroying healthy tissue in its way, and continues growing.[2]

Cancers are classified into five major groups: carcinomas, sarcomas, lymphomas, leukemias, and adenomas. Tumors in the visceral tissues of the body are carcinomas, whereas sarcomas are located in cartilage, connective tissue, bone, muscle, fat, and other supportive tissue. Lymphatic cancers are in the immune system and lymph nodes. Leukemias start off in the bone marrow and usually gather in the bloodstream. Finally, adenomas are cancers in glandular tissues, such as the adrenal gland, the thyroid, and the pituitary gland.[3]

CAUSES OF CANCER

In the developed world, nearly 20 percent of cancer cases are caused by infectious diseases, such as hepatitis B and C. Other causes can include genetic defects, smoking, drinking alcohol, obesity, a lack of physical activity, and a poor diet. Substances that can directly damage DNA and promote or aid cancer development are called carcinogens. Examples of carcinogens are asbestos, tobacco, and solar and gamma radiation.[4]

Almost 30 percent of people with chronic HBV develop chronic liver disease, which may lead to liver cancer. Some evidence shows that a coinfection with hepatitis D increases the chance of developing cancer. A small fraction of HCV patients who develop cirrhosis will form malignant tumors. The average time of developing liver cancer after infection with hepatitis C is about twenty-eight years. Liver cancer in HCV patients can be due to factors such as heavy alcohol use, age, gender, coinfection with HIV or hepatitis B, and cirrhosis.[5]

Responsible for around 75 percent of liver cancers, hepatocellular carcinoma is formed by hepatocytes that become malignant. Hepatoblastoma is another type of liver cancer that is formed in preliminary liver cells that have not yet fully matured. This malignant tumor is rare and usually occurs in children, accounting for almost 90 percent of liver cancer cases in individuals under the age of fifteen. Cholangiocellular cystadenocarcinoma and cholangiocarcinoma, making up less than 10 percent of liver cancer cases, are malignant tumors in the bile duct. Rhabdomyosarcoma and leiomyosarcoma are cancers of the liver muscles. Other rare types include carcinoid tumors, carcinosarcomas, and lymphomas. A lot of cancers in the liver spread from other parts of the body to the liver and are not in fact liver cancers.[6]

SIGNS AND SYMPTOMS OF CANCER

Signs and symptoms vary depending on the size, location, and spread of the cancerous growth. Certain cancers might be felt through the skin as lumps in the cancerous area. Melanoma (skin cancer) presents as changes in moles or warts on the skin. Brain tumors can affect cognitive function; as a result, these tumors can engineer the immediate signs and symptoms of hepatitis. Pancreatic cancer only presents symptoms at a later stage, when it has grown enough to start pushing against nerves nearby and causing pain. Prostate cancer causes more or less frequent urination because it changes bladder function. Because of its interference with normal hormone function, cancer can exhibit tiredness, anemia, excessive sweating, weight loss, and fever.[7]

Cancer significantly affects cells. Cells are expected to grow in a controlled manner; however, if the genetic formation of the cells is affected, the control on composition is lost. The cells then collect, grow, and form irregularly and spread in the affected person's body. Cancerous cells can form in any tissue and may cause severe physical disorders. With liver cancer, the liver can no longer produce much-needed enzymes for the body, barring its essential functions. Liver cancer can also produce deep ulcers in the liver that cause it to slowly rot. Patients can feel a strong pain in the upper abdominal region. Digestive difficulties occur if the cancer is untreated.[8]

DIAGNOSING LIVER CANCER

Diagnosing liver cancer is done with a number of imaging modalities. These include computer tomography (CT), magnetic resonance imaging (MRI), and ultrasound. Chemicals that can be found in the blood of people with cancer, called tumor markers, help diagnose and monitor the progress of the cancer. Increased levels of alpha-fetoprotein in a person's blood may indicate hepatocellular carcinoma or intrahepatic cholangiocarcinoma.[9]

TREATMENT

Surgical removal of a tumor and healthy tissue around it, also called segmental or surgical resection, is in most cases the treatment of choice for patients with noncirrhotic livers. For cirrhotic livers, surgical resection can pose a great risk of liver failure. More than 50 percent of patients who undergo removal surgery have a five-year survival rate. Unfortunately, in 70 percent of cases, recurrence of cancer happens because of initial tumor spread or new tumors.[10]

A liver transplant is also an option for people who fit the "Milan criteria." This criteria states that a patient may have up to three lesions under three centimeters and/or one lesion smaller than five centimeters but have no extrahepatic manifestation and no vascular invasion. Because hepatocellular carcinoma is often detected at a late stage, 60 to 70 percent of individuals are not be eligible for transplant or any far-reaching surgery.[11]

The only nonsurgical treatment that may be a cure is percutaneous ablation, a therapy in which certain chemicals are injected into the liver and/or the liver is subjected to temperature extremes using lasers, microwaves, radiofrequency ablation, or cryotherapy. Radio frequency ablation has shown the most potential. One of the major downsides with this treatment is the inability to treat tumors close to blood vessels or other organs (e.g., the liver) due to the heat-sink effect that comes with this treatment. Radiotherapy is rarely used to treat these types of cancers because of the liver's intolerance to radiation.[12]

PREVENTION

The first rung in the prevention of liver cancer is to moderate exposure to its risk factors; the most effective preventative is the hepatitis B vaccination. At this time, there are no vaccines available for hepatitis C. However, one can limit the transmission of the virus by screening high-risk individuals and promoting safe injection practices. Also, reducing obesity, diabetes, and alcohol abuse can help prevent liver cancer.[13]

A second level of prevention is for those with a dangerous hepatitis infection. If a cure of the viral infection is not possible, patients must actively manage it to prevent carcinogenesis. Interferon therapy, for example, decreases the risk of liver cancer. The last step of prevention is reducing the risk of recurrence through chemotherapy or drugs.[14]

ANALYSIS

Hepatitis B and hepatitis C are the main direct and indirect causes of liver cancer. Eighty percent of hepatocellular carcinoma cases, the most prevalent of liver cancers, occur in patients with HBV or HCV. The viral infection can cause issues such as massive inflammation, fibrosis, and cirrhosis, which significantly increases the risk of hepatocellular carcinoma. There are, however, hepatitis C sufferers whose livers develop cancer in the absence of cirrhosis. Furthermore, it is believed that the core protein of the HCV virus is the primary malefactor in the development of liver cancer. This protein might be responsible for interfering with the normal function of a tumor suppressor gene, or it may also be an impediment in the natural process of cell death. These factors allow liver cells to replicate unchecked, thereby leading to malignant liver tumors.[15]

19

TYPES OF LIVER DISORDERS

Located in the upper-right section of the abdomen, the liver is a vital element in the body's digestive system. It is the largest internal organ and is responsible for metabolizing and storing most nutrients absorbed by the intestine. The liver is also in charge of producing proteins and detoxifying the blood by removing harmful chemicals and processing them to be excreted later.[1]

A liver disorder is defined as any disturbance of liver function. Most liver disorders share a few common symptoms such as nausea, vomiting, jaundice, and abdominal pain in the upper-right quadrant. Patients can also experience weakness, fatigue, weight loss, and other symptoms specific to each type of liver disease.[2] Apart from hepatitis, there are in excess of one hundred other types of known liver disorders. The most common are:[3]

- alcoholic liver disease,
- cirrhosis,
- fascioliasis,
- fatty liver disease,
- primary liver cancer,
- primary biliary cirrhosis,
- primary sclerosing cholangitis,
- centrilobular necrosis,
- liver failure,
- hemochromatosis,

- Budd–Chiari syndrome,
- Wilson's disease, and
- Gilbert's syndrome.

There are also many pediatric liver diseases, such as alpha-1 antitrypsin deficiency, Alagille syndrome, biliary atresia, and progressive familial intrahepatic cholestasis. Many of the rampant liver disorders in the world have been linked to viral hepatitis. An untreated viral infection can have a domino effect that leads to cirrhosis, liver failure, liver cancer, and more. In order to prevent these diseases, hepatitis sufferers should get screened and vaccinated against hepatitis B, especially if they are at high risk. Patients already diagnosed with viral hepatitis (B or C) should start antiviral treatment as soon as possible to avert further complications.[4]

COMMON LIVER DISORDERS

Alcoholic liver disease is the main source of liver cirrhosis in the United States. Also called Laennec's cirrhosis, alcoholic liver disease generally advances after years of alcohol abuse. The greater the amount of alcohol ingested and the longer the periods of excessive consumption, the higher the chances of developing this disease. Aside from the symptoms shared with other liver disorders, alcoholic liver disease can also cause dry mouth, confusion, loss of appetite, fever, and ascites, which is excessive fluid between the abdominal organs and the membrane lining the abdomen. Some patients with the disease may also exhibit hallucinations, agitation, abnormally light or dark coloration of the skin, and short- or long-term memory loss. In the first phases, this disease can appear as fat accumulation in the liver, also known as fatty liver disease. In some individuals, alcoholic liver disease at this stage also causes an inflammatory reaction to this change of fat in liver cells, known as alcoholic hepatitis. While these two conditions are considered reversible, later stages of the disease may produce cirrhosis and fibrosis, which are usually irreversible. It is imperative to discontinue alcohol consumption as part of alcoholic liver disease therapy. A midrange caloric, high-carbohydrate diet to suspend any uncontrolled protein breakdown is also helpful. Milk thistle has been noted to help improve liver function, more so in milder forms of the disease.[5]

Cirrhosis is characterized as the formation of scar tissue (fibrosis) in place of dead liver cells. Cirrhosis has many different causes, but the most common are viral hepatitis, fatty liver disease, and alcoholic liver disease. This disease has a wide variety of symptoms, some a direct cause of failing liver cells, others as a result of conditions like portal hypertension. A few direct symptoms include ascites, gynecomastia (increased size of the breast glands in men), hypogonadism (decrease in sex hormones), and spider angiomata (vascular lesions). The absence of symptoms does not eliminate the possibility of cirrhosis. A number of complications can arise from cirrhosis, such as hepatocellular carcinoma, hepatic encephalopathy, and esophageal variceal bleeding. Treatment is aimed at preventing complications because cirrhosis itself cannot be reversed. If an advanced stage is reached, then a liver transplant is the only solution.[6]

Fatty liver disease is a disorder where fat accrues in liver cells through the process of steatosis. Although causes for fatty liver disease vary, the most prominent culprits are excessive alcohol intake and obesity. Approximately 70 percent of obese people develop nonalcoholic fatty liver disease. This liver disorder can be either asymptomatic or have vague symptoms that are easily confused with other health issues. If left untreated, this liver disorder can lead to steatohepatitis, then cirrhosis, and end-stage liver disease. Treatment consists of lifestyle changes, such as cutting alcohol consumption; avoiding drugs that can harm the liver; treating lipid disorders; and taking multivitamins, antioxidants, and milk thistle products.[7]

Primary liver cancer, also called hepatocellular carcinoma, is the most pervasive cancer of the liver, usually a result of viral hepatitis or cirrhosis. Other causes may include hemophilia, hemochromatosis, type 2 diabetes, and Wilson's disease. Symptoms of liver cancer can be yellowing of the skin, bruising from blood clotting, bloating from abdominal fluid, and abdominal pain. Treatment options depend on a number of factors, especially the tumor's stage and size.[8]

Fascioliasis, also known as liver rot, is a disease caused by two parasitic worms called fasciola hepatica, commonly known as liver fluke, and fasciolagigantica. The disease is more common in animals, but recently it has emerged in humans. An estimated 2.5 million people around the world are infected with this parasite, and 180 million are at risk. Infection in humans occurs by ingesting certain plants that may contain the parasites, such as lamb's ear, watercress, dandelion leaves, or spearmint. Raw liver dishes and untreated fresh water can also be a source of infection. The parasitic infection has four stages: incubation, acute, latent, and chronic. The acute, or invasive, stage is when the mechanical destruction of liver tissue begins and symptoms emerge. These include ascites, anemia, high fever, abdominal pain, and gastrointestinal disturbances. The most effectual treatment for humans is the drug triclabendazole.[9]

Hemochromatosis, also called iron overload, is a disorder leading to abnormal levels of iron accumulation. This surplus of iron surfaces in the liver, pancreas, or heart and can develop into cirrhosis, liver failure, and liver cancer. Hemochromatosis is a genetic disorder but can also be caused by repeated blood transfusions. Routine treatment consists of regular bloodletting therapy (scheduled phlebotomies).[10]

Similar to hemochromatosis, Wilson's disease is a genetic liver disorder that consists of high levels of copper buildup in tissue. The main areas of copper accumulation are the brain and the liver. Consequentially, there are a number of neuropsychiatric and liver-disease-related symptoms. Treatments include a low-copper-intake diet combined with medication that either prevents copper absorption or helps remove excess copper from the body. A liver with hepatitis is susceptible to all the liver disorders covered here.[11]

ANALYSIS

If a person with HCV or HBV has already developed another liver disorder, then therapy should be carefully designed to challenge the hepatic infection. The last resort is a liver transplant if damage is otherwise irreversible. Transplants require a compatible donor, which can be difficult to find, and it also poses the possibility of death. Transplants also require the patient to fit specific criteria (i.e., the Milan criteria), with the objective of reducing the risk of disease and physical damage to the new liver.[12]

20

RELATED NONHEPATIC DISORDERS

Mental disorders cannot be diagnosed exclusively by brain imaging or by workups in a medical laboratory; they are primarily determined by an individual's behavior. Over the years, differentiating physical disorders from mental disorders has proven to be formidable in law and medicine. Doing so requires a deep analysis of unresolved arguments in both psychology and philosophy. Some believe that mental disorders are accentuated by physical ailments, such as hepatitis, though tests have not yet confirmed such a phenomenon.[1]

There are mental conditions that only *reportedly* originate directly from tissue pathology. Psychiatrists do believe that all or some mental disorders are the result of some sort of physical vagaries in the brain. Certain physical disorders can also be made worse or even caused by mental illness. However, physical disorders are treated physically, and people react to these diseases and treatments differently. Health-care workers, however, take a holistic perspective: They examine social and mental factors contributing to diseases like hepatitis.[2]

Physical disorders may be classified into three broad groups. Prenatal physical disorders are acquired before birth; they may be caused by substances or a disease that harmed the mother before or during the pregnancy. Perinatal physical disorders are acquired at the time of birth; this may be due to lack of oxygen, premature birth, and brain damage. Postnatal physical disabilities are acquired after birth and may be due to infections, accidents, or other illnesses.[3]

The three groups of physical disorders can further be divided into another three subsections: impairments of vision, mobility, and hearing. Mobility impairment affects body limbs and the coordination of various organs. It may be caused by old age or a broken skeletal structure. Visual impairments are caused by minor or severe vision injuries and may be corrected through surgery. Hearing impairment may lead to partial or permanent deafness. Some physical disorders are known to cause seizures, chronic pain, fatigue, and lack of sleep, among other conditions. As physical disorders come in different forms and have various effects on people, they also are caused by a myriad of factors.[4]

Asthma is a physical disorder that affects a person's air passage. It affects breathing and most often affects sleep. Constant wake-ups at night when having an attack can cause fatigue. Patients with asthma find it difficult to take part in commonplace activities, such as sports, which can make them feel socially isolated and unmotivated.[5]

A recent study firmly links diabetes to depression and anxiety. One in every six patients diagnosed with type 2 diabetes experiences anxiety. One in every four people with type 2 diabetes is depressed. With type 1 diabetes, one in seven and one in five people experience depression and anxiety, respectively.[6]

Chronic pain is a prolonged pain that lasts beyond the time in which procedures are expected to heal. It often happens after trauma or surgery. If not attended to, chronic pain is known to affect a person's routine day-to-day activities, exercise, sleep, work, lifestyle, and social interactions.[7]

Myalgic encephalitis is a condition that causes inexorable fatigue that may last for long periods, almost always over six months. Initially, it was thought only to affect educated young adults, but it has been proven to affect people of all ages from all walks of life. The condition is more prevalent in women than men. It is caused by viral infections (like hepatitis), immune reactions, and environmental toxins, to name a few. Other causes are being reviewed, including endocrine-metabolic dysfunction.[8]

Epilepsy is characterized by seizures, from rigorous to little or nearly unnoticeable shaking. Epilepsy occurs more frequently with unknown cause, while some people develop epilepsy following brain tumors, brain injuries, and alcohol and drug misuse. Epileptic seizures are caused by abnormal and excessive nerve cell activity within the brain.

About 70 percent of epileptic seizures can be controlled by medication; however, people who do not respond to medication may consider dietary changes or neurostimulation as an alternative treatment.[9]

The occurrence of autistic spectrum disorder is not fully understood, but experiments show that both the environment and genes play a role. Autism is characterized by significant impairment at work, socially, and in day-to-day activities. Its symptoms may be seen at the early stages of childhood and is characterized by a withdrawal from social interaction and difficulty communicating.[10]

Dyspraxia is a coordination problem in both adults and children; in some cases, speech is also affected. It is a lifelong condition that affects each patient differently and may change depending on life experiences and environmental demand. Symptoms include poor balance, lack of rhythm when dancing, poor posture, poor manipulative skills, and continuous and repetitive talk. People with dyspraxia tend to get stressed and have difficulty sleeping, low self-esteem, phobias, addictive behavior, and emotional outbursts. Adults with dyspraxia tend to experience more problems than children.[11]

ANALYSIS

Regardless of whether someone was suffering a disorder before being diagnosed with hepatitis or if the disorder was caused by the disease, the best course of action is to seek treatment for both conditions as fast as possible. Treatment for mental disorders and other nonhepatic matters may be support groups, medication, and therapy or a combination of all three.[12]

IV

Resolutions

21

NATURAL APPROACHES FOR HEPATITIS

A standard treatment for hepatitis is not proven effective for every patient, so it is understandable to look for reliable alternative treatments. Before discussing the efficacy of the alternative treatment, patients and caregivers need to consider the possible side effects. Experts strongly suggest not taking any medicines, vitamins, or supplements without obtaining a prescription. Unforeseen reactions to pills, whether natural or pharmacological, should be kept in mind.[1]

TREATING HEPATITIS NATURALLY

Some natural treatments, such as acupuncture, massage, and yoga, have no direct role in treating hepatitis but can be used in conjunction with standard treatment to relieve the pain and side effects of standard treatment. Although some natural biologics are not scientifically proven to be effective in treating hepatitis, they are relatively safe in comparison with conventional (allopathic) medicine, and hence the risk of side effects is minimal. Natural herbs have been reported to improve the immune system, and some herbs are reported to improve the functions of the liver. If patients are physiologically unresponsive to standard treatment, they often choose to take alternative medicines and have reported restored liver functions.[2]

There are many natural treatments available to treat hepatitis C, but this chapter focuses only on those that have been well-studied. Some

Chinese natural treatments do exist for treating hepatitis B, but because of the lack of research, they are excluded here.[3]

Milk thistle is a well-studied antioxidant and anti-inflammatory herb for treating hepatitis C. A small but noteworthy study reports that milk thistle can decrease the level of inflammation in the liver for patients who are nonresponsive to the standard treatment. Nonetheless, milk thistle is *not always* effective in treating hepatitis. When coupled with interferon, silymarin, a vital ingredient of milk thistle, may considerably decrease the level of inflammation. Side effects of milk thistle are limited; hence, safety regarding the usage of milk is not an issue. The exact efficacy of milk thistle in treating hepatitis is still unclear.[4]

Licorice root has been reported to increase liver functions, whether taken alone or with other herbs. However, taking licorice root in greater quantity is reported to have such side effects as high blood pressure and high potassium loss. Licorice root cannot be taken with certain heart medications and heart conditions, such as high blood pressure, heart disease, or any other chronic disease, thus it is important to consult a specialist.[5]

As the name implies, thymus extract is derived from the thymus gland of a cow. It has been speculated that taking thymus extract can increase immune system functioning; however, it is not recommended as a supplement, for it may lead to contamination and may pose a threat to the normal functioning of certain organs. There are also reports suggesting that thymus extract can jettison the work of blood platelets. At this stage of very limited research, thymus extract is not recommended.[6]

Other natural treatments, such as acupuncture, massage, yoga, and traditional Chinese medicine (TCM), have been suggested as an alternative to standard hepatitis treatment. None of these treatments have been proven to effectively suppress any form of hepatitis, but when they are taken in conjunction with standard treatments, the disease may improve. There are very few studies that suggest that TCM can cure hepatitis B. Acupuncture and massage can help to relieve pain caused by standard treatment. Yoga and other breathing workouts do not have any direct role in the treatment of hepatitis, but they may improve the confidence of the patient. Professional massage may also improve the morale of hepatitis sufferers.[7]

DIET IN HEPATITIS MANAGEMENT

Healthy eating has many benefits for fighting hepatitis, and any treatment plan is incomplete without a proper diet. As the disease progresses, loss of appetite becomes more acute and can lead to malnourishment. By lightening strain on the liver, healthy eating buys the liver more time to fight the disease. The immune system is also freed to better deal with hepatitis. Although the effects of the diet may not be immediate one will find their body and soul drastically improved in the long run.[8]

Diets can vary from person to person; hence, a specialist may suggest one diet for one patient and a different diet for another. A basic or minimalistic diet with a high percentage of protein, carbohydrates, and low-fat food is usually suggested for hepatitis patients. For anorexic patients, such a diet can help greatly. All patients should consume easily digestible food that is low cholesterol, low fat, and high fiber in four small meals each day to aid digestion. Wheat, gluten, dairy products, and junk foods should be avoided, as they take more time to digest. It is also strongly advised to avoid smoking and especially drinking alcohol for at least six months. Green and yellow vegetables are particularly healthy for the liver. Homemade juice is preferable to store-bought, as those from the shop contain too much sugar. In some hepatic postsurgery cases, the hospital nutritionist may recommend a diet high in proteins and carbohydrates, such as those rich in eggs, fish, and chicken, for a quicker recovery of liver tissue.[9]

Sugars, including artificial sweeteners, should be avoided, as they may inflame hepatitis C symptoms and incite diabetes. People infected with hepatitis have a greater chance of suffering from diabetes, and controlling blood sugar levels decreases the risk. [10]

Those with hepatitis can adopt more advanced dietary habits, such as adopting fruit meals, to help them conquer their disease-related issues. If one is in a hurry, fruits, such as apples or bananas, are great meals. Bananas are nutritious, and with other ingredients, hepatitis patients can customize bananas to their personal tastes.[11]

Finally, milk can be valuable for overall nutrition, though nondairy products are highly recommended for hepatitis patients. While some hepatitis patients do not prefer plain milk, there are chocolate mixes or similar powders that can be added to it to increase the intake of minerals essential for health. Some vitamins, such as vitamin K, vitamin D, vitamin E, and vitamin B complex, are very important for chronic hepatitis patients. Patients should consult their health-care professionals first to get a proper dosage of these vitamins and minerals.[12]

ANALYSIS

It is easy to surmise that all-natural products and herbs are safe, but that is not the case. Alternative treatments can have multiple side effects, some of which may result in serious consequences. It is highly suggested to consult a specialist before taking any natural product or herbs.[13]

22

EXERCISE FOR HEPATITIS PATIENTS

Physical exercise or workout is intensified activity that improves or maintains the well-being of the body and the soul. Exercise plays a crucial role in preventing and treating chronic diseases. Although most exercises have no direct role in treating a disease, it can improve the morale and health of a person to effectively fight disease. In order to understand which exercises are helpful to hepatitis patients, it is wise to know the origins of exercise as a remedy itself.[1]

HISTORY OF EXERCISE

Exercise is not confined to the twenty-first century, but it is now prevalent due to the obesity epidemic. Although the origin of exercise is not known, traditionally physical activity, such as hunting and gathering, was required for people to survive. At least five thousand years ago, the ancient civilizations of China and India introduced physical exercises such as yoga, kung fu, and gymnastics. Yoga uses breathing exercises, stretching, and meditation to improve physical and spiritual well-being. Developed by Hindu priests, many yoga exercises may be difficult for ordinary individuals.[2]

Prominent ancient Greek physicians, such as Herodotus and Hippocrates, were very concerned with health. In ancient Greece, gymnastics was often taught with music because it was thought to relieve the soul from pain while the former mitigated physical pain. Exercise was also prevalent in ancient Roman civilization: All individuals after adolescence were given military training to protect the nation.[3]

Exercise began to spread among Western countries only in the beginning of the eighteenth century. Although most exercise forms were borrowed from China, India, and other countries, today, modern exercise is a result of Western origin as older exercise forms have been lost with time. Once civilization transitioned from hunting to agriculture and technology, physical activity decreased.[4]

EXERCISE FOR HEPATITIS PATIENTS

Exercise should only be completed under the guidance of a physician who is knowledgeable about hepatitis. Exercise and sufficient rest helps hepatitis patients relieve stress and be happy. When exercising, one should avoid newly painted areas, as paint fumes, thinners, and household cleaning products can affect the liver. Moreover, a hygienic environment is essential at the gym.[5]

Physical exercise is recommended for hepatitis patients for two major reasons: One is to stay within the healthy weight range. This prevents other dangerous complications, such as high blood pressure, heart disease, and diabetes, that are often associated with hepatitis. The second reason is to alleviate symptoms of hepatitis. Hepatitis is usually accompanied by pain that requires pain killers. Exercise is suggested to relieve stress on the liver, as the use of several painkillers can degrade the liver.[6]

Aside from diet, proper exercise is needed to maintain a healthy weight. Regular exercise can reduce BMI, and experts suggest that even mild physical exercise can help reduce weight. Being in shape and within a healthy BMI range can prevent most complications associated with any liver disease. A healthy BMI also prevents fatty substance buildup in the liver, which can degrade the liver's condition and increase inflammation. To achieve results in relatively less time, hepatitis patients may try intensive cardiovascular drills. To make things more exciting, one can even try mountain biking and cycling. It is best to consult a physician before beginning a rigorous exercise regimen, as medical history may affect the degree of intensity allowed.[7]

HEALING THROUGH EXERCISE

Although the medical field has made substantial progress, the standard treatment for hepatitis patients is still not perfect, as it has many potential side effects. It is important to keep in mind that patients cannot fight hepatitis with only drugs and treatment; exercise is necessary for their bodies, as well as souls, when dealing with the healing process. Scientists believe that patients who regularly exercise can better tolerate the risks of standard hepatitis treatment than those who do not.[8]

Breathing exercises, such as yoga and meditation, have no direct role in relieving liver pain associated with hepatitis, but they can improve the morale and concentration of hepatitis patients. Hepatitis patients need more sleep than ordinary people do. As yoga and meditation relieve stress, these exercises can also be helpful for better sleep.[9]

ANALYSIS

Research suggests that exercise not only reinforces liver health, but also makes one more responsive to treatment for any liver disease. If a patient is not obese, then an aerobic exercise regimen should suffice to improve liver health. If the patient is obese, then appropriate steps must be taken, even if the hepatitis is abated. Exercise can improve the immune system; hence, the liver is protected from disease. Exercise also improves stamina and blood circulation, both of which increases the body's ability to fight disease. Thus, exercise is a crucial part of a treatment plan for a healthy liver.[10]

23

PHARMACOLOGICAL APPROACHES TO HEPATITIS

Medications comprise a massive business worldwide, whether pharmacological or alternative. In America alone, billions are expended on pharmacological pills, herbs, and other dietary supplements. Understandably, when hepatitis patients seek treatment, they subsequently prefer the most effective and safest methods at their disposable. In addition to natural remedies, hepatitis specialists look toward pharmacological routes because they are perceived in the medical community as more potent and effective.[1]

Patients with liver failure and comas are afforded antibiotics, such as neomycin or metronidazole. Due to the drastic fall in production of serum bilirubin, corticosteroids are recommended. Prednisolone is prescribed for anywhere from five to thirty days as the usual course. Hepatitis patients also can be prescribed very low doses of acetaminophen (a marginal pain reliever and fever reducer), as it is not hepatotoxic (does not harm the liver easily). If a patient complains of restlessness, then the doctor can prescribe narcotic drugs, such as phenobarbital or diazepam.[2]

Antipruritics can be prescribed to patients if they complain of itching. Calamine lotion containing phenol and cholestyramine is used to moderate pruritus in patients with cholestatic jaundice. Ultraviolet light treatment may also be effective. Moreover, chronic hepatitis patients may be given prednisolone every twenty-four hours during the initial stage. The goal is to reduce the dosage after about two weeks and then continue gradually reducing the dosage until the patient reaches a maintenance dose in the following weeks. In addition to corticosteroid therapy, a person with hepatitis may receive azathioprine once a day. If the patient is unresponsive to combined prednisolone and azathioprine, then cyclosporine may be taken every twenty-four hours.[3]

For chronic hepatitis B patients, antiviral therapy is recommended. To inhibit formation of harmful DNA molecules, nucleoside analogues may be prescribed. Some patients convert from HBeAg-positive to HBc-antibody drugs, which may contain famciclovir, adefovir, lobucavir, and lamivudine.[4]

A hepatitis patient could be given cytokine therapy to address the hyperactivity of interferon alpha, beta, gamma, and interleukin. Lymphoblastoid and recombinant interferon-alpha have promising results. A combination of prednisolone initially, followed by interferon-alpha therapy, may be recommended to an individual with chronic hepatitis B. Famciclovir or lamivudine with viral-suppression therapy may be prescribed to patients with chronic hepatitis B for several years.[5]

Adefovir, entecavir, lamivudine, telbivudine, or tenofovir are in order if the hepatitis patient is suffering from liver cirrhosis. Danoprevir has had promising results in treatment. For individuals with nonviral hepatitis, the physician will eliminate the destructive elements or substance. Hyperventilation or induced vomiting can be used to flush out and clean the stomach, and such patients may be prescribed corticosteroids for an immune system boost.[6]

DRAWBACKS OF PHARMACOLOGICAL APPROACHES

When someone is weakened by hepatitis, the typical side effects of prescription medications include fever, body and muscle aches, nausea, headaches, vomiting, ulcers, skin rashes, and poor appetite. The mental impact can get worse in such scenarios, with otherwise-healthy people experiencing poor sleep, insomnia, anxiety, or depression as a consequence of hepatitis drugs. Furthermore, patients with cirrhosis cannot use interferon. Instead, they may be prescribed more direct antivirals, such as adefovir, entecavir, lamivudine, telbivudine, or tenofovir. Some drugs and medicines may cause serious side effects in the treatment of hepatitis C. Symptoms include chest pain, shortness of breath, vision changes, and thyroid pain. These serious side effects may greatly affect the patient. In such cases, patients must immediately contact their caregivers and health-care professionals so they can be placed under medical observation.[7]

ANALYSIS

To reap the benefits of pharmacological medication, one must confront the risks and consider the unwelcome side effects as well as the helpful results. To secure the most out of treatment, hepatitis patients should not hesitate to speak with pharmacists, nurses, physicians, or other health-care professionals about physiological sensitivities to pharmacological strategies.[8]

24

HEPATITIS AND SURGERY

Surgery can produce lasting results when a patient commits to lifelong alterations in exercise and diet. Surgical patients by and large enjoy a better quality of life after their operations. They also witness a reduction in health problems that justified the surgery in the first place. Patients suffering from acute viral hepatitis, chronic hepatitis, or alcoholic hepatitis are susceptible to surgical errors, thus hepatitis emergencies should be dealt with immediately. Surgery can be a favorable option in such regard.[1]

SURGICAL PROCEDURES FOR HEPATITIS

Preliminary surgical options for a patient suffering from hepatitis B do not exist. If the patient presents themselves with advanced liver damage due to hepatitis and the disease is life threatening, a surgeon may recommend a liver transplant. A transplant is the only option for a patient with fulminant hepatitis, wherein there is sudden liver failure associated with hepatitis B. A person with elevated blood alcohol level may not be eligible for a donation, as continuing an unhealthy lifestyle that would wound the liver again is likely.[2]

A liver transplant is surgery used to remove a severely infected and diseased liver and replace it with one donated from another person. The orthotropic transplantation is the most adaptable standard technique used for the liver transplant. The procedure replaces the affected liver with the liver provided by the donor in the same anatomical location. This may be the only option for patients with acute liver failure or at a critical stage of liver disease. Multiple anesthesia experts, such as anaesthesiologists, nurse anesthetists, and even rotational surgeons, are usually involved in the surgery. Depending on the condition of the patient and results, the transplantation may go on for hours. Plenty of disconnections and reconnections of abdominal and hepatic tissues with multiple anastomoses and joints are done for a successful transplant. Liver support therapy might be specified to bridge the time until transplantation. Radiofrequency ablation of liver tumors can also bridge treatment while patients await a liver transplant.[3]

Many liver transplants use nonliving donors. For an infant or a small child who requires a liver transplant, portions of an adult's liver can be transplanted. Recent developments make split-liver transplantation a possibility. Through this process, one liver is used for two recipients. Living donor transplant innovations have also reshaped the field of organ transplant. Thanks to living donor transplantation, parts of a living individual's liver is removed and used as an allograft to replace the diseased part of the recipient's liver. In this case, the recipient can be released from the hospital within five to seven days with a speedy recovery.[4]

Liver transplantation surgery is divided into three phases. The first stage, the hepatectomy phase, is the removal of the diseased liver. The second phase is the anhepatic phase, and the third phase is the postimplantation phase. The hepatectomy phase is the division of all ligamentous attachments to the liver, common bile duct, and hepatic artery and vein. Ice cold storage holds blood that will replenish the blood lost from the donor's liver. Then the hepatic, portal, lower vena cava, and other blood vessels are rewired.[5]

Immunosuppressive drugs are used most commonly following transplant operations. A transplant patient who used to have hepatitis prior to the surgery may receive corticosteroids and tacrolimus or cyclosporine and mycophenolatemofetil. Studies suggest promising results and better responses to tacrolimus when compared with cyclosporine following the first year of liver transplantation surgery.[6]

DRAWBACKS TO HEPATITIS-RELATED SURGERY

Liver rejection may occur any time after the transplant surgery. There are three types of rejections that may occur after liver transplants:[7]

1. **Hyperacute rejection:** Happens within only minutes or hours after liver transplantation. Hyperacute rejection is a B-cell-facilitated rejection.
2. **Acute rejection:** T-cell mediated. Cytotoxicity and cytokines are involved in acute rejection. Immunosuppressive agents are the primary targets during acute rejection. Acute rejection can occur within days or weeks of the liver transplant.
3. **Chronic rejection:** Occurs a year after liver transplant. There are no clear explanations for chronic rejection, but acute rejection is a strong forecaster.

Per laboratory data, the side effects and other drawbacks to liver transplant include abnormal AST, ALT, GGT, and prothrombin time ammonia levels; abnormal concentration of albumin; unusual bilirubin level; and irregular blood glucose levels. Jaundice, bruising and bleeding propensity, and encephalopathy are also potential side effects.[8]

ANALYSIS

Even nontransplant surgeries performed for liver cancer following extreme hepatitis can result in a replacement tumor after the cancerous part is removed. This is especially true if the remaining liver contains the underlying viruses for a very long time. Surgery can improve mobility for hepatitis patients as liver pain recedes. Nonetheless, if the damage is not severe, then the patient could be better off with noninvasive resolutions instead of risking a dismal outcome from surgery.[9]

25

MENTAL ASPECTS

Psychological dilemmas are on the rise for individuals with chronic hepatitis. Several factors such as alcohol abuse and low social support may contribute to this upsurge. The psychological effects and changes in the quality of life for viral hepatitis patients are common and should be treated with urgency. Regardless of the severity of hepatitis, patients who also have cirrhosis need improved treatment and psychological education due to the greater number of problems than others. This, patients must address the social factors that may be affecting their health.[1]

PSYCHOLOGICAL STATUS OF THE HEPATITIS PATIENT

Mental health issues can severely limit performance and quality of life. Individuals with hepatitis should be treated in a manner that eases mental stress. The most important duty falls on health-care providers, because they must address psychological trauma without exacerbating the situation. Psychological trauma is never rectified without effort, as issues may resurface in unpredictable ways. Unfortunately, some may see hepatitis patients differently from others. This perception can trouble patients, making some feel incompetent.[2]

Hepatitis involves sensitive issues that should be treated with greater importance. Since depression is one of the most troubling aspects for hepatitis patients, one should heal in an environment that also addresses mental stress. One way of mitigating depression is by taking a vacation to ensure a calm state of being.[3]

STAYING JOYFUL WHILE DEALING WITH HEPATITIS

Achieving long-term, stable happiness may be one of the toughest challenges for any liver disease patient. However, proper nutrition can also act as a source of happiness. It may be difficult for caretakers to give proper nutrition to the hepatitis patients, but they can provide meals that cater to the patient's taste and make the patient feel that he is being cared for. Caregivers can also experiment with new recipes. It is important to incorporate a balanced diet, *gradually* adding new foods to a patient's daily meals.[4]

DEALING WITH THE STRESS: AT HOME AND IN THE OFFICE

Patients are often stressed when they find out they have hepatitis. Nevertheless, patients must maintain a healthy balance between household and office tasks. Hepatitis is contagious, so the chances of a critically infected hepatitis patient actively engaged in an occupational setting with many others in close proximity are very slim. If the hepatitis is mild, a healthy balance is attainable for everyone.[5]

Hepatitis-related stress is understandable but not negligible. People with hepatitis can listen to music at home or in the office to relax. They can also connect with others to temporarily disregard their own issues. Finally, exercise can help reduce stress.[6]

ANALYSIS

Continued stress only harms one's state of mind in the long term. Most stress is due to the mental pressure of coping with the disease. However, patients can retain some of their normal, stress-free lives. It is possible to focus on things other than the illness. If one has the determination, then the disease can be fought, be it at home or in the office.[7]

26

ADJUSTING TO LIFE AS A HEPATITIS PATIENT

Everyone has a few bad habits. Bad habits only promote the negative, which is why it is important for hepatitis patients to initiate better habits now rather than later. Good habits can help a patient be healthier and live longer. Therefore, one should ditch harmful actions as soon as possible and engage in a lifestyle to furnish what is required for healing.[1]

Lifestyle change is important for improving health because it helps ensure a longer life. The lifestyle changes that really make a difference are those that achieve balance. Everyone, including caregivers, must support the lifestyle changes to accomplish a working reality.[2]

LIFESTYLE AND MEDICAL CARE

Patients may visit their hepatitis physicians two, three, or more times a month as situations demand. Physicians can closely monitor the status of patients and their livers to take preventive actions. Charts should be updated at the clinic at every visit. As prescribed by the doctor, one should get vaccinated for hepatitis A and B to stay shielded against infection. Sometimes it is best for the patient not to take exceptionally high doses of vitamins or other supplements, as some are potential toxins.[3]

Hepatitis sufferers must understand the disease in order to achieve a positive lifestyle. Patients should monitor what they eat and research what should be in their diet to be healthy and moderate liver damage. Moreover, one should strictly follow the diet plan referred by the hepatitis expert (see chapter 21). They should avoid ingesting any food or liquid that may affect the liver. It is also helpful to keep fit.[4]

It is possible to live healthily and actively if the hepatitis patient follows proper medical treatment prescribed by the physician and adopts an auspicious lifestyle. Hepatitis patients can make even seemingly insignificant changes to their lifestyles and improve their physical and mental states.[5]

PERSONAL LIFESTYLE CHANGES

The function of the liver is to filter toxins that are potentially dangerous for the body out of the blood supply. The consumption of alcohol, tobacco products, and other drugs affects the capacity of this large organ. Hepatitis patients looking to make a change in their lifestyle should always keep that in mind.[6]

If a hepatitis patient works at a chemical plant, then continuing the job is not advised. Fumes generate toxins that are dangerous for the liver and liver functions. Extended exposure may eventually lead to liver failure. Family members and caregivers of hepatitis patients can use eco-friendly cleaners and toiletries; many contemporary cleaners are acid-based and can produce fumes that are dangerous for people with hepatitis. A strong and healthy liver may effectively filter these toxins, but a diseased liver does not possess the same fervor. It is important to address these small details to prevent chronic hepatitis, which may lead to liver failure.[7]

Viral hepatitis patients must prevent transmitting the disease to their loved ones, since it spreads fast within tissues and organs. Direct contact with infected body fluids, such as blood and semen, swiftly spreads hepatitis. Infected donated blood can cause hepatitis C. Unprotected sex with a virally infected partner may cause hepatitis B. Sexual partners need to be tested immediately; if they are found to be negative, then they must be treated at once. It is recommended to avoid sharing toothbrushes, razors, needles, nail clippers, and earrings.[8]

The following are common practices to prevent hepatitis:[9]

- Do not eat overpreserved food. Only eat fresh food or food that has been in the refrigerator for a short while.
- Use only filtered or boiled water.
- Hands must be kept clean as much as possible. Wash hands prior to eating and after toilet use.
- Remain current on vaccinations.
- Do not share drug equipment, such as needles. Use brand-new needles and syringes each time.
- Do not eat expired foods.
- Do not eat food from cans with leaks or holes.
- Get plenty of rest, and relieve stress through meditation.

ANALYSIS

The lifestyle changes that one decides to make now are essential for a brighter tomorrow. Hepatitis sufferers can wake up to an improved and much healthier body on all fronts. One needs to make amendments to his lifestyle oneself; no one can change a person's life on his behalf. Lifestyle change is, of course, much more than just a better diet and exercise. A wholesome lifestyle makes it all come together in the end.[10]

27

ADVANCEMENTS IN HEPATITIS RESEARCH

Clinical research is the systematic collection of clinical data and its analysis, evaluation, and interpretation, performed with the goal of contributing to advancements in the scientific field. Research in hepatology contributes immensely to the health industry. Additionally, discovering how human cells work is important in the prevention and treatment of not only hepatitis but other diseases and conditions as well. Clinical research is proof of how science guides development of miracle drugs and scientific breakthroughs for hepatitis. Such cause-and-effect relationships date back to the early seventeenth century when the discovery of the inner workings of blood in animals paved the way for major findings. Thus, the lasting presence of clinical research in all subjects, including hepatitis, was set off.[1]

BENEFITS OF CLINICAL RESEARCH

Clinical research enhances understanding of cell structures and functions, including in the liver. It also promotes an understanding of the organisms that cause liver diseases, how they compromise human cells, how human cells react to them, and what can be done to augment natural healing.[2]

Disease-causing microorganisms change constantly, which means that liver histologists must develop better medicine to tackle them at the tissue level. Clinical research in collaboration with epidemiology supports the development of different drugs, along with testing and safety checks. Related inquiry also helps pharmacists to discover new ingredients, both natural and synthetic, for different types of drugs. Therefore, the research field streamlines the manufacturing of medicine.[3]

There are medical conditions that cannot be cured but can easily be managed with therapy. Scientific and clinical research is used to devise more efficient therapies by improving on existing forms of therapy. Doctors and other medical professionals are also able to improve on different practices used in the medical field. There are numerous health risks that one simply might not realize but that threaten the lives of all. Clinical studies help to determine these risk factors and ultimately formulate successful ways to mitigate these risks.[4]

ADVANCES IN PREVENTION RESEARCH

The main prevention technique involved in the management of hepatitis is providing society with a safe and clean water supply. Strict care of sewage disposal is important. It is also crucial to treat infected individuals to prevent an epidemic, thus, isolation is necessary.[5]

For more technical investigations, there is prevention research. Current treatment choices are confined to alpha-interferon alone or integrated with ribavirin. Sadly, these methodologies have moderately poor viability and an unfavorable reaction profile. New studies have yielded up-to-the-minute methodologies for prophylactic and helpful immunizations, interferon's enhanced pharmacokinetic qualities, and novel medications to hinder the capacity of three noteworthy viral proteins: protease, helicase, and polymerase.[6]

The HCV RNA genome, especially the IRES component, is often misused as an antiviral target using antisense particles and reactant ribosomes. Albeit not exhaustive, this survey condenses the latest discoveries in this quickly evolving field.[7]

Research proves that immunization is powerful for a long time. The Centers for Disease Control and Prevention (CDC) suggests that all infants, teens, and adults in danger of contamination be inoculated. Vaccination of young individuals (one to eighteen years old) is comprised of a few dosages of concentrated immunization. Adults need a booster six to twelve months after the first immunization. Protected and viable immunizations safeguard against hepatitis B for fifteen years and potentially longer.[8]

ADVANCES IN DIAGNOSTIC RESEARCH

Diagnosis of hepatitis is completed by a doctor in a lab or in clinical research facilities. Hepatitis C is spread through direct contact with contaminated blood. Transmission through other bodily fluids is rare, but this is still under scientific scrutiny. One should have his blood checked for the hepatitis B antigen (HBsAg), which generally shows up in the bloodstream six to twelve weeks after the onset of disease. If the results are positive, the person has hepatitis B. Then, specialists must conduct further tests to ascertain whether the virus is a recent or older infection. If a patient does not respond negatively to HBsAg, then they are safe from future infection of hepatitis B.[9]

Specialists will first check for hepatitis C antibodies (hostile to HCV), which generally take seven to nine weeks to show up postinfection. A positive result means that one currently has the infection or it has recently cleared. If the immune system is weakened, then it may take more time to create hepatitis C antibodies, or there may not be any at all. If the first test is positive, then the specialist will check for the virus itself (hepatitis C RNA). If this is also positive, then hepatitis C is definitely present.[10]

ADVANCES IN HEPATITIS LONG-TERM THERAPY

There have been recent headways in therapy research. Treatment of more than one hundred patients with the hepatitis B-e antigen yielded improvements. These patients were on average thirty-four years old and were mostly Asian males. After five years in the study, the mean (average) changes in serum hepatitis were noticeable.[11]

Around 25 percent of patients with chronic hepatitis C will face cirrhosis; some of these patients will see an enlargement of the liver or liver failure. This is one reason scientists are working fervently to find a vaccine for hepatitis C. Long-term treatment for hepatitis C is a blend of alpha interferon or pegylated interferon (antiviral and invulnerable fortifying medications) and ribavirin. Alpha interferon is given by infusion three times each week; pegylated drugs are given by infusion just once every seven days.[12]

Around half of patients administered these infusions improve, but numerous patients do not respond well to treatment. A study on fifty patients with chronic hepatitis C who did not respond to mixed treatment or who could not withstand the side effects of interferon or pegylated interferon treatment, underwent liver biopsies to address their present liver conditions. Some began an outpatient single-medication treatment with ribavirin, given orally twice a day with a dosage based on the patient's body weight. They were instructed to return for normal checkups and blood tests every two to eight weeks for the duration of the study. After six months, the drug was ceased or balanced, depending on the findings of the subject's liver blood tests. A positive response was documented if half or more of the introductory liver protein (almandine aminotransferase, ALT) was diminished. Owing to developments in long-term clinical therapy, scientists now know without a doubt that a positive response to treatment has happened if chemicals in the liver return to ordinary levels.[13]

When it was found that chimpanzees and apes are the only species except humans that can contract hepatitis viruses, hepatitis research was conducted on these animals. The conditions for such research were life-threatening, as humans working with animal subjects could also contract the pathogen. They were also able to demonstrate that the modulator of a molecule called GS-9620 has a receptor recognized by immune system cells. Another group of scientists have suggested that all forms of hepatitis are utterly curable, proof of much clinical progress.[14]

Clinical science evolves to improve, save, or extend life. This is what makes scientific medicine different from technology. Inevitably, however, these two entities often contradict each other. Advanced clinical research is the foundation for the breakthrough or discovery of a cure for all forms of hepatitis.[15]

ANALYSIS

Without solid clinical science, any new drug or medical device crumbles like a house of cards. This is why it is imperative that extensive scientific testing be performed to establish a treatment's efficacy. It is not enough just to analyze medical documentation. Clinical research must pick through the findings with a fine-toothed comb. Sooner or later, the benefits of clinical research in the field of hepatology will yield results. For now, immortality is a pipe dream, but clinical research might soon make this impossible dream a reality.[16]

28

COLLECTIVE EFFORTS

Society can develop initiatives that hold the government and health-care providers accountable for the state of health in any country. This is an effective way to persuade governments and private hepatitis health-care providers to (1) maintain the highest levels of standards, (2) provide high-quality services and medicine, (3) ensure that all members of the society have access to affordable health care, and (4) increase their commitment to continually improving health-care provisions. The health-care industry exceedingly depends on the government, private practitioners, and facilities to thrive. This calls for the private and public health sectors to work collaboratively in order to provide quality health care to all populations. The following highlights how governments and society can achieve this within the scope of hepatitis.[1]

GOVERNMENTS AND REDUCTION OF HEPATITIS

Governments of individual countries need to step up their efforts in fighting this disease. Because vaccination provides 99 percent immunity in some strains of hepatitis A and B, it is crucial that governments and their acting agencies are committed to making vaccinations available to all. Government support of large-scale vaccination has helped control once-widespread hepatitis, but it is only possible with coordinated efforts.[2]

There are also a number of chemical drugs, toxic substances, and other components that cause specific hepatitis-related ailments. Governments can be indispensable for identifying such causes, cataloguing their regional spread, and discovering how to expel these viruses. Without a specific framework and guidelines for community-level medicine, it is impossible to effectively control the potential destruction. The government must also raise awareness; provide medical aid; and include the information about the disease, its symptoms, and its prevention in the educational curriculum. The involvement of government agencies in the fight against the disease will not only cut medical costs related to the disease but also will provide more extensive care.[3]

Various national and international institutions are battling this disease in their own ways, with whom the government of any country can coordinate. Governments can help strengthen these institutions by supporting their agenda to bring the disease to an end. Government agencies everywhere must stand at the forefront of the fight against the disease.[4]

The government in collaboration with the private sector can engage in diverse scientific and health research to enhance the medical field. Nonprofit government organizations (NGOs) with donors can provide funding and resources for research, while society provides experts, test subjects, and data related to all liver conditions. Medicines, therapies, and equipment could then be tested and certified by government and independent agencies to make them ready for application.[5]

One of the greatest ways to effectively use the health resources in a country is to educate the citizens on available services, where they can get these services, their expected cost, and available payment methods. Society can collaborate with governments to support educational forums. Governments control through regulations activities in any field and the care for chronic illnesses; hepatitis is no exception. To ensure good practices, governments should collaborate with society to develop regulations and standards that promote health and well-being. Governments should always allow society to scrutinize regulations and suggest improvements before they are enacted. This inclusive process also ensures that society feels part and parcel of the process and is more likely to comply with these regulations.[6]

HOW NONMUNICIPAL BUSINESSES AND CORPORATIONS CAN HELP

Governmental intervention alone cannot relegate the growing annual deaths due to hepatitis. Various businesses and corporations have to be directly *and* implicitly involved in the collective effort against the disease. Many businesses partially responsible for the disease (e.g., by producing unhygienic items) have to eradicate their own internal sources of the problem. Drug manufacturers must provide written warnings on packaging for prescriptions, as they may be the cause of various forms of hepatitis. Moreover, corporations can provide financial assistance or establish free vaccination days. Because the fight against this massive killer is also a social fight, any health and medical institution can get involved.[7]

The bout with this disease can improve immensely if businesses and agencies are involved internationally. Encouraging and supporting volunteers globally can produce collective change. Social organizations and clubs all over the world can play a vital role by raising awareness at the grass-roots level.[8]

PATIENTS SUPPORTING EACH OTHER

Apart from all these collective efforts, the most important and effective care is patient self-care. The primary focus should be on prevention of disease rather than its care. However, for those who have already contracted the disease, direct care in hospitals and support from others with the same disease can be helpful. Sharing information on late and early symptoms and medical care is valuable to patients. Such suggestions are substantial and often parallel to those of medical professionals.[9]

Former patients can help by writing blogs, articles, and correspondence with heath-support groups. They can also help by visiting the hospitals and meeting patients individually. This may not be possible in all cases, but such visits collectively can raise awareness. The support provided can also serve as a psychological boost for hepatitis patients in immediate need. When unified with patient self-care and familial care, the support can help a patient to accept the disease.[10]

Patients should not be negligent and must be proactive in fighting hepatitis. Those who have contracted it and fought it triumphantly have precious information to share about the disease itself, its symptoms, and its cure. Everyone who has gone through this can help future patients by being resources, thereby lowering the mortality of hepatitis. Finally, sometimes a person cannot explain his anomalies to a medical team, but a presence of another patient can make it work.[11]

ANALYSIS

Governments as well as patients can help hepatitis sufferers. The collective result of these efforts is extraordinary and will only further the eradication of hepatitis, giving birth to a healthier society. Thus, in a collective fight against this disease, each stakeholder must step up their efforts against this threat. Governments need to involve businesses and other social institutions. Of course, these efforts will not bear fruit without the involvement of the patients themselves and those who are at risk. The fight against hepatitis is not a singular fight. This disease is a global problem, and the battle against it should be a concerted effort.[12]

V

Homestretch

29

HOPE, PATIENCE, CONFIDENCE, AND RESPONSIBILITY

The importance of hope in health care cannot be underestimated. When patients are hopeful that they will get better, they will strive for quality medical care and will keep taking medications according to their doctor's instructions. Hope also ensures that patients with chronic illnesses like hepatitis get the best care even in their last days on earth.[1]

PATIENCE WHEN DEALING WITH HEPATITIS

If one expects something to happen, one must have patience. Hepatitis sufferers can take the initiative to read more while resting during the progression of treatment. A dedicated person cannot be impatient for a cure. He knows that only patience will lead to the goal or destination. Such people keep calm and maintain a clear mind to achieve the true reward at the end, which is a healthy liver. The person who has patience can easily handle upcoming unhappy situations. Rome was not built in a day, and hepatitis does not kill instantly. Therefore, patients should not let negative emotions take over.[2]

CONFIDENCE WHEN DEALING WITH HEPATITIS

The benefits of confidence when suffering with hepatitis are many. While hope is important, those who are suffering from hepatitis should not just hope for an instant cure. Remaining confident is an active process, but it can also improve a patient's ability to cope with other hardships. No gifts in life are straightforward without hope, patience, and confidence. Confidence can be attainable to some but invisible to others. Some individuals feel a quick onset of illness, with nausea, yellowed skin, fatigue, darkened urine, and abdominal pain. These symptoms might stay for weeks at a time but will eventually disappear. A confident patient understands this.[3]

RESPONSIBILITY WHEN DEALING WITH HEPATITIS

A hepatitis patient needs to accept their role in order to effectively conquer the disease. The first responsibility is to provide accurate information to medical practitioners so that patients can receive accurate diagnoses and the most suitable treatment. This includes medical history, symptoms, medications, existing medical conditions, and any other details that health-care professionals may deem necessary. Second, patients must follow the recommended medical plan faithfully to ensure that they get well and that the liver does not develop resistance to the drugs. Likewise, the patient has a responsibility to respect medical providers and other patients. Hepatitis sufferers should use a medical facility with respect so that it can be comfortabe for others who follow. This includes hospital furniture, equipment, fixtures, and utensils. Patients should also make sure they pay their bills from medical practitioners in a timely manner.[4]

Hepatitis viruses are infectious. Although people can fight off this disease within few months, it has some drawbacks for the human body. When patients get frustrated and want to resolve the problem immediately, they should see a doctor rather than self-prescribing. In some countries, many individuals are illiterate and have traditions rooted in the belief of superstitions. As a result, they often refuse to go to a conventional doctor for treatment, which threatens the health of the entire population. Hepatitis can remain dormant in one's body for many years and become active at unpredictable times. Physician-based treatment should last until the patient is cured. Pathology tests may provide proof of infection but not evidence of liver damage, so hepatitis sufferers can be contagious and transmit this disease to other people.[5]

ANALYSIS

Hope, patience, confidence, and responsibility ensure that everyone involved can handle anything regarding hepatitis. Having these qualities also improves self-worth, which in turn improves how liver disease patients relate with caregivers around them. It is, therefore, important for people with hepatitis to remain resolute during their ordeal and to promote a culture of hopefulness in those around them.[6]

GLOSSARY

acute hepatitis: liver inflammation or hepatitis for only a short period of time (six months or less).
albumin: abundant plasma protein that is synthesized by the liver.
alexia: a disorder associated with reading due to problems of internally identifying sounds.
alkaline phosphatase: protein enzyme synthesized by the liver, especially in the presence of bile-duct obstruction.
alpha-fetoprotein (AFP): an elevated level of this protein indicates possible liver cancer (AFP levels are also elevated during pregnancy).
anhepatic phase: the stage of liver transplantation when the diseased liver is removed and the patient is briefly without a liver.
antibody: also known as immunoglobulin, which neutralizes certain pathogens.
antigen: a biological molecule that stimulates an immune system response.
ascites: condition where the peritoneal cavity or the abdomen has free fluid, indicating chronic liver disease.
autoimmune hepatitis: formerly called lupoid hepatitis, where the body's immune system attacks the liver cells.
bile: one of the fluids created and released by the liver and stored in the gallbladder.
bilirubin: a product of the red blood cells' chemical breakdown, an indicator of liver disease, hemolytic anemia, and bile-duct obstruction.
body mass index (BMI): the number achieved by dividing the weight of a person in kilograms by height in meters squared.
cell: the fundamental functional and structural component of all living things.
Centers for Disease Control and Prevention (CDC): a national public health agency concerned with research and prevention of disease outbreaks.
chronic: illness that persists or lasts for a long period, more than three months.
chronic active hepatitis: an advanced form of hepatitis where the liver injury is widespread and the liver has been infected for more than six months.
chyme: partly digested food that travels from the stomach to the small intestine.
cirrhosis: the result of long-term liver damage, which is scarring and permanent impairment of the liver cells.
contagious: a disease that can be transferred from one person to another through direct or indirect contact.
cure: relieving an individual of his symptoms entirely or to heal and restore to good health.
dehydration: the result of a body loss of too much water, sometimes because of illnesses affecting the gastrointestinal tract.

delirium: an unexpected state of confusion that is severe and with rapid deterioration in brain functioning.
diagnosis: the exact identification of an illness and the nature of a certain disease.
dysbetalipoproteinemia: increased levels of LDL, unhealthy lipoproteins, cholesterol, phospholipids, and triglycerides.
dyspraxia: a speech coordination problem seen in both adults and children.
emergency department: a medical treatment room in any hospital specializing in emergency medication and acute treatment.
endemic: an illness commonly found in a specific region or population.
enzyme: a substance that speeds up the chemical reactions in the body.
epidemic: an increase in the spread of a disease in a short period of time.
epilepsy: a condition characterized by seizures, which causes an individual to shake uncontrollably.
epithelium: the outermost layer of the skin that protects all open surfaces of the body.
fatigue: a feeling of severe tiredness and decreased energy to do everyday activities.
fibrosis: the development of abnormally excessive fibrous connective tissue in the liver.
gastroenterologist: a medical doctor who specializes in the liver and the gastrointestinal tract.
genome: the genetic information or material of an organism.
GI tract: the gastrointestinal tract, also known as the digestive system.
HAV: hepatitis A virus.
Havrix: hepatitis A vaccine.
HBsAg: hepatitis B surface antigen that indicates hepatitis B infection.
HBV: hepatitis B virus.
HCV: hepatitis C virus.
headache: pain felt above the eyes, ears, or at the back of the head.
hepatectomy phase: the removal of the diseased liver.
hepatic portal vein: a blood vessel responsible for moving blood from the GI tract to the liver.
hepatitis: several types of infectious conditions of the liver that causes inflammation.
hepatitis A: liver inflammation due to the hepatitis A virus, usually transmitted via the fecal–oral route or through drinking or eating contaminated water or food.
hepatitis B: liver inflammation due to the hepatitis B virus, usually transmitted through blood and other infected body secretions (semen, vaginal discharges, saliva, breastmilk).
hepatitis C: liver inflammation due to the hepatitis C virus, also transmitted through infected blood, and the common cause of lymphoma and liver cancer.
hepatitis D: liver inflammation due to the hepatitis D virus, which only occurs in the presence of hepatitis B.
hepatitis E: liver inflammation due to the hepatitis E virus, usually transmitted through drinking contaminated water.
hepatitis G: inflammation of the liver in which the symptoms are very mild.
hepatitis X: an unknown and undefined virus that causes inflammation of the liver.
hepatocytes: liver cells.
hepatologist: medical doctor who specializes in the diagnosis and treatment of the liver.
hepatomegaly: liver enlargement.
hormones: the chemical messengers of the human body released by endocrine glands.
hygiene: set of practices that prevents disease and preserves health.
immune: an individual or organism that is safeguarded against certain infections.
immune system: an organ system that defends the body against diseases.
immunity: the condition in which the body has reached a good homeostasis to fight microorganisms, bacteria, and viruses that results in strong biological defense.
infection: the infiltration and rapid increase of the number of microorganisms, including viruses and bacteria in the body.
inflammation: a localized reaction of the body indicated by pain, redness, swelling, and warmth.

interferon: also known as signaling proteins that are produced and released by host cells in the body that aid in strengthening the immune system.
jaundice: the yellowish color of the sclera and skin when there is too much bilirubin in the bloodstream.
Kupffer cells: specialized macrophages in the liver responsible for the elimination of microbial toxins, endotoxins, and the like.
Licorice (liquorice) root: a plant said to improve the functions of the liver if taken alone or with other herbs.
liver: the largest internal organ, located in the upper-right abdomen.
liver disease: any identified liver disorder.
liver failure: a life-threatening condition where the liver is totally damaged and incapable of performing important functions, such as synthesizing and metabolizing.
liver function test (LFT): a laboratory examination of liver enzymes in blood.
lobule: a tiny lobe.
lymphocytes: a type of white blood cell responsible for vital immune responses.
metabolism: a series of chemical reactions that generates energy to run processes in the body.
milk thistle: an antioxidant and anti-inflammatory herb.
myalgic encephalitis: a condition that causes unrelenting fatigue that may last for long periods, almost always over six months.
nausea: the urge to vomit.
pain: unpleasant sensation associated with tissue damage.
pandemic: an illness that affects a high portion of the population over a wide geographical region or all over the world.
pegylated interferon: an antiviral and anticancer component of medications.
portal hypertension: the increased pressure in the portal venous system, indicating obstruction due to liver disease.
postimplantation phase: liver transplantation stage after the liver is implanted in a recipient.
prognosis: the predicted outcome of a disease or the rate of recovery.
protein: a large molecule created from amino acids and used as a tissue-building source by the body.
prothrombin time: laboratory examination of the blood's clotting time, a good indicator of the liver's overall function.
RNA virus: virus with ribonucleic acid as its genetic material.
rubella: also known as German measles, a mild infection that lasts seven to ten days.
scientific method: the processes of discovery and demonstration characteristic of or necessary for scientific evaluation.
serum: colored liquid that separates with clotted blood.
sign: a feature of a disease that is subjective to the outside observer.
silymarin: a vital ingredient of milk thistle, when coupled with interferon, may considerably decrease the level of inflammation.
spider nevi: visible growth of branched capillaries in the skin.
surface antibody positive (IgG): a molecule or indicator of an individual who was previously infected with the hepatitis B virus and has since recovered.
sustained virologic response: when the hepatitis C virus cannot be detected in the blood while the individual is undergoing treatment.
synthesize: to create something chemical.
thymus extract: derived from the thymus gland of a cow that is speculated to increase immune system functioning.
vaccination: administration of a vaccine for the purpose of stimulating immunity to a particular virus or other microorganism.
vaccine: substance created from weakened or killed microorganisms that stimulates immunity.
viral: pertaining to a virus.
virus: a small, very harmful biological agent that reproduces itself inside cells.

NOTES

PREFACE

1. Wu JF, Chang MH. Natural history of chronic hepatitis B virus infection from infancy to adult life: The mechanism of inflammation triggering and long-term impacts. *J Biomed Sci.* 2015; 22(1): 92.

2. Pybus OG, Thézé J. Hepacivirus cross-species transmission and the origins of the hepatitis C virus. *Curr Opin Virol.* 2015; 16: 1–7.

3. Strauss SM, Astone JM, Des Jarlais DC, Hagan H. Integrating hepatitis C services into existing HIV services: The experiences of a sample of U.S. drug treatment units. *AIDS Patient Care and Standards.* 2005; 19(2): 78–88.

4. Weissberg JI, Andres LL, Smith CI, et al. Survival in chronic hepatitis B: An analysis of 379 patients. *Ann Intern Med.* 1984; 101(5): 613–16.

5. Rothman AL, Morishima C, Bonkovsky HL, et al. HALT-C trial group. *Hepatology.* 2005; 41(3): 617–25.

6. Poordad F, Dieterich D. Treating hepatitis C: Current standard of care and emerging direct-acting antiviral agents. *J Viral Hepat.* 2012; 19(7): 449–64.

7. Lee HC. Acute liver failure related to hepatitis B virus. *Hepatol Res.* 2008; 38(Suppl 1): S9–S13.

8. Cuthbert JA. Hepatitis A: Old and new. *Clin Microbiol Rev.* 2001; 14(1): 38–58.

9. Langer BC, Frösner GG, von Brunn A. Epidemiological study of viral hepatitis types A, B, C, D, and E among Inuits in West Greenland. *J Viral Hepat.* 1997; 4(5): 339–49.

10. Liao BL, Lin SW, Shi HY, He HL, Zhang JS, Cai WP. Clinical feature analysis of 334 chronic hepatitis B patients coinfected with hepatitis E virus. *Zhonghua Gan Zang Bing Za Zhi.* 2015; 23(9): 697–99.

11. Shah HA, Abu-Amara M. Education provides significant benefits to patients with hepatitis B virus or hepatitis C virus infection: A systematic review. *Clin Gastroenterol Hepatol*. 2013; 11(8): 922–33.

12. Geier DA, Geier MR. Hepatitis B vaccination and adult associated gastrointestinal reactions: A follow-up analysis. *Hepatogastroenterology*. 2002; 49(48): 1571–5.

I. INTRODUCTION: IMPORTANCE OF LIVER HEALTH

1. Ramadori G, Moriconi F, Malik I, Dudas J. Physiology and pathophysiology of liver inflammation, damage and repair. *J Physiol Pharmacol*. 2008; 59(Suppl 1): 107–17.

2. Rui L. Energy metabolism in the liver. *Compr Physiol*. 2014; 4(1): 177–97.

3. Murphy JD, Hattangadi-Gluth J, Song WY, et al. Liver toxicity prediction with stereotactic body radiation therapy: The impact of accounting for fraction size. *Pract Radiat Oncol*. 2014; 4(6): 372–77.

4. Ramadori G, Moriconi F, Malik I, Dudas J. Physiology and pathophysiology of liver inflammation, damage and repair. *J Physiol Pharmacol*. 2008; 59(Suppl 1): 107–17.

5. Schroeder B, McNiven MA. Importance of endocytic pathways in liver function and disease. *Compr Physiol*. 2014; 4(4): 140–17.

6. Merion RM, Schaubel DE, Dykstra DM, Freeman RB, Port FK, Wolfe RA. The survival benefit of liver transplantation. *Am J Transplant*. 2005; 5(2): 307–13.

7. Norman K, Pirlich M. Gastrointestinal tract in liver disease: Which organ is sick? *Curr Opin Clin Nutr Metab Care*. 2008; 11(5): 613–19.

8. Chi H, Haagsma EB, Riezebos-Brilman A, van den Berg AP, Metselaar HJ, de Knegt RJ. Hepatitis A related acute liver failure by consumption of contaminated food. *J Clin Virol*. 2014; 61(3): 456–58.

9. Perri GA. Ascites in patients with cirrhosis. *Can Fam Physician*. 2013; 59(12): 1297–99; e538–40.

10. Tindale WB, Barber DC, Smart HL, Triger DR. Liver blood flow: Non-invasive estimation using a gamma camera. *Proc Inst Mech Eng H*. 1992; 206(2): 99–103.

11. Çelik Ö, Kahya MC, Nazıroğlu M. Oxidative stress of brain and liver is increased by wi-fi (2.45GHz) exposure of rats during pregnancy and the development of newborns. *J Chem Neuroanat*. 2016; 75(B): 134–39.

12. Pawlotsky JM. Pathophysiology of hepatitis C virus infection and related liver disease. *Trends Microbiol.* 2004; 12(2): 96–102.

13. Kmieć Z. Cooperation of liver cells in health and disease. *Adv Anat Embryol Cell Biol.* 2001; 161: iii–xiii, 1–151.

2. ANATOMY OF HEPATITIS

1. Juza RM, Pauli EM. Clinical and surgical anatomy of the liver: A review for clinicians. *Clin Anat.* 2014; 27(5): 764–69.

2. Pierce L. Anatomy and physiology of the liver in relation to clinical assessment. *Nurs Clin North Am.* 1977; 12(2): 250–73.

3. Ghosh SK. Human cadaveric dissection: A historical account from ancient Greece to the modern era. *Anat Cell Biol.* 2015; 48(3): 153–69.

4. Hoe CM, Wilkinson JS. Liver function: A review. *Aust Vet J.* 1973; 49(3): 163–69.

5. Gissen P, Arias IM. Structural and functional hepatocyte polarity and liver disease. *J Hepatol.* 2015; 63(4): 1023–37.

6. Triger DR. Physiological functions of the liver. *Br J Hosp Med.* 1979; 22(5): 424, 429–30, 432.

7. Sato M, Suzuki S, Senoo H. Hepatic stellate cells: Unique characteristics in cell biology and phenotype. *Cell Struct Funct.* 2003; 28(2): 105–12.

8. Iwamura K. Clinical aspects of bile acid metabolism in liver diseases. *Tokai J Exp Clin Med.* 1982; 7(1): 7–29; Williams CN. Bile-acid metabolism and the liver. *Clin Biochem.* 1976; 9(3): 149–52; Read AE. Clinical physiology of the liver. *Br J Anaesth.* 1972; 44(9): 910–17; Grand RJ, Ulshen MH. Clinical and physiological abnormalities in hepatic function. *Pediatr Clin North Am.* 1975; 22(4): 897–928; Rothuizen J. Important clinical syndromes associated with liver disease. *Vet Clin North Am Small Anim Pract.* 2009; 39(3): 419–37.

9. Sakamoto Y, Kokudo N, Kawaguchi Y, Akita K. Clinical anatomy of the liver: Review of the 19th meeting of the Japanese Research Society of Clinical Anatomy. *Liver Cancer.* 2017; 6(2): 146–60.

3. PHYSIOLOGY OF HEPATITIS

1. Rui L. Energy metabolism in the liver. *Compr Physiol.* 2014; 4(1): 177–97.

2. Seeger C, Mason WS. Molecular biology of hepatitis B virus infection. *Virology.* 2015; 479–80: 672–86.

3. Stocum DL. Regenerative biology and medicine. *J Musculoskelet Neuronal Interact*. 2002; 2(3): 270–73.

4. Stanger BZ. Cellular homeostasis and repair in the mammalian liver. *Annu Rev Physiol*. 2015; 77: 179–200.

5. Abd El-Kader SM, Al-Jiffri OH, Al-Shreef FM. Liver enzymes and psychological well-being response to aerobic exercise training in patients with chronic hepatitis C. *Afr Health Sci*. 2014; 14(2): 414–19.

6. Pawlotsky JM. Pathophysiology of hepatitis C virus infection and related liver disease. *Trends Microbiol*. 2004; 12(2): 96–102.

7. Luo JC, Hwang SJ, Chang FY, et al. Simple blood tests can predict compensated liver cirrhosis in patients with chronic hepatitis C. *Hepatogastroenterology*. 2002; 49(44): 478–81.

8. Yanchuk PI, Athamnah SM, Reshetnik EM, Levadyanska JA, Nikitina NO, Veselsky SP. Role of serotonin in the regulation of respiration and bile secretory function of the liver. *Fiziol Zh*. 2015; 61(2): 102–10.

9. Bhoday HS, Jain NP, Kaur H, Pannu HS, Singh P, Sood A. To study the prevalence of impaired glucose tolerance in patients with hepatitis C virus related chronic liver disease. *J Clin Diagn Res*. 2015; 9(3): OC16–20.

10. Felmlee DJ, Hafirassou ML, Lefevre M, Baumert TF, Schuster C. Hepatitis C virus, cholesterol and lipoproteins: Impact for the viral life cycle and pathogenesis of liver disease. *Viruses*. 2013; 5(5): 1292–324; Bilzer M, Roggel F, Gerbes AL. Role of Kupffer cells in host defense and liver disease. *Liver Int*. 2006; 26(10): 1175–86.

11. Kmieć Z. Cooperation of liver cells in health and disease. *Adv Anat Embryol Cell Biol*. 2001; 161: iii–xiii, 1–151.

12. Fausto N. Liver regeneration and repair: Hepatocytes, progenitor cells, and stem cells. *Hepatology*. 2004; 39(6): 1477–87.

4. DIGESTIVE HEALTH

1. Leslie T, Pawloski L, Kallman-Price J, et al. Survey of health status, nutrition and geography of food selection of chronic liver disease patients. *Ann Hepatol*. 2014; 13(5): 533–40.

2. Johnstone C, Hendry C, Farley A, McLafferty E. The digestive system: Part 1. *Nurs Stand*. 2014; 28(24): 37–45; Hendry C, Farley A, McLafferty E, Johnstone C. The digestive system: Part 2. *Nurs Stand*. 2014; 28(25): 37–44.

3. Ojeda A, Moreno LA. Pain management in patients with liver cirrhosis. *Gastroenterol Hepatol*. 2014; 37(1): 35–45; Keller U, Szinnai G, Bilz S, Berneis K. Effects of changes in hydration on protein, glucose and lipid metabolism in man: Impact on health. *Eur J Clin Nutr*. 2003; 57(Suppl 2): S69–74.

4. Wang ZK, Yang YS. Upper gastrointestinal microbiota and digestive diseases. *World J Gastroenterol*. 2013; 19(10): 1541–50.

5. Casanova J, Bataller R. Alcoholic hepatitis: Prognosis and treatment. *Gastroenterol Hepatol*. 2014; 37(4): 262–68.

6. Nogaller AM. Effectiveness of health resort treatment of chronic hepatitis and liver cirrhosis with lipotropic factors as diet supplement. *Sov Med*. 1958; 22(10): 65–74.

7. McKenna O, Cunningham C, Gissane C, Blake C. Management of the extrahepatic symptoms of chronic hepatitis C: Feasibility of a randomized controlled trial of exercise. *Am J Phys Med Rehabil*. 2013; 92(6): 504–12.

8. Han P, Yang L, Huang XW, et al. A traumatic hepatic artery pseudoaneurysm and arterioportal fistula, with severe diarrhea as the first symptom: A case report and review of the literature. *Medicine (Baltimore)*. 2018; 97(7): e9893.

9. Takahashi H, Shigefuku R, Yoshida Y, et al. Correlation between hepatic blood flow and liver function in alcoholic liver cirrhosis. *World J Gastroenterol*. 2014; 20(45): 17065–74.

10. Petrasek J, Iracheta-Vellve A, Saha B, et al. Metabolic danger signals, uric acid and ATP, mediate inflammatory cross-talk between hepatocytes and immune cells in alcoholic liver disease. *J Leukoc Biol*. 2015; 98(2): 249–56.

11. Gershon MD. 5-Hydroxytryptamine (serotonin) in the gastrointestinal tract. *Curr Opin Endocrinol Diabetes Obes*. 2013; 20(1): 14–21.

12. Johnstone C, Hendry C, Farley A, McLafferty E. The digestive system: Part 1. *Nurs Stand*. 2014; 28(24): 37–45.

5. CIRCULATORY SYSTEM HEALTH

1. Borzecki A, Zółkowska D, Sieklucka-Dziuba M. Life style and the risk of development of circulatory system diseases. *Ann Univ Mariae Curie Sklodowska Med*. 2002; 57(1): 426–32.

2. Teragawa H, Hondo T, Amano H, Hino F, Ohbayashi M. Adverse effects of interferon on the cardiovascular system in patients with chronic hepatitis C. *Jpn Heart J*. 1996; 37(6): 905–15.

3. Tsukada K, Suematsu M. Visualization and analysis of blood flow and oxygen consumption in hepatic microcirculation: Application to an acute hepatitis model. *J Vis Exp*. 2012; (66): e3996.

4. Ioannou GN, Morishima C, Yu L. Sex difference in liver-related mortality and transplantation associated with dietary cholesterol in chronic hepatitis C virus infection. *Br J Nutr*. 2015: 1–9.

5. Pawlotsky JM. Pathophysiology of hepatitis C virus infection and related liver disease. *Trends Microbiol*. 2004; 12(2): 96–102.

6. Marzouk D, Sass J, Bakr I, et al. Metabolic and cardiovascular risk profiles and hepatitis C virus infection in rural Egypt. *Gut*. 2007; 56(8): 1105–10.

7. Gielen S, Laughlin MH, O'Conner C, Duncker DJ. Exercise training in patients with heart disease: Review of beneficial effects and clinical recommendations. *Prog Cardiovasc Dis*. 2015; 57(4): 347–55; Heran BS, Chen JM, Ebrahim S, et al. Exercise-based cardiac rehabilitation for coronary heart disease. *Cochrane Database Syst Rev*. 2011; (7): CD001800.

8. Martínez-Esparza M, Tristán-Manzano M, Ruiz-Alcaraz AJ, García-Peñarrubia P. Inflammatory status in human hepatic cirrhosis. *World J Gastroenterol*. 2015; 21(41): 11522–41.

9. Cueni LN, Detmar M. The lymphatic system in health and disease. *Lymphat Res Biol*. 2008; 6(3–4): 109–22.

10. Alitalo K. The lymphatic vasculature in disease. *Nat Med*. 2011; 17(11): 1371–80.

11. Onji M, Michitaka K, Yamauchi Y. Morphometric analysis of lymphatic and blood vessels in human chronic viral liver diseases. *Am J Pathol*. 1998; 153(4): 1131–37.

12. Borzecki A, Zółkowska D, Sieklucka-Dziuba M. Life style and the risk of development of circulatory system diseases. *Ann Univ Mariae Curie Sklodowska Med*. 2002; 57(1): 426–32.

6. HISTORY OF HEPATITIS

1. Ashfaq UA, Idrees S. Medicinal plants against hepatitis C virus. *World J Gastroenterol*. 2014; 20(11): 2941–47.

2. Westbrook RH, Dusheiko G. Natural history of hepatitis C. *J Hepatol*. 2014; 61(1 Suppl): S58–68; Chen PC, Corciova FC, George G, Hsieh WC, Tinica G. Prevalence of post-operative morbidity risk factors following cardiac surgery in patients with chronic viral hepatitis: A retrospective study. *Eur Rev Med Pharmacol Sci*. 2015; 19(14): 2575–82.

3. Lawrence SP. Advances in the treatment of hepatitis C. *Adv Intern Med*. 2000; 45: 65–105.

4. Ali AH, Carey EJ, Lindor KD. Primary biliary cirrhosis. *Lancet*. 2015; 386(10003): 1565–75; Hashim MJ, Khan G. Burden of virus-associated liver cancer in the Arab world, 1990–2010. *Asian Pac J Cancer Prev*. 2015; 16(1): 265–70.

5. Dalton HR, Froud OJ, Harris N, et al. The natural history of autoimmune hepatitis presenting with jaundice. *Eur J Gastroenterol Hepatol*. 2014; 26(6): 640–45.

6. Starzl TE, Iwatsuki S, Van Thiel DH, et al. Evolution of liver transplantation. *Hepatology*. 1982; 2(5): 614–36.

7. Carver DH, Seto DS. Hepatitis A and B. *Pediatr Clin North Am*. 1974; 21(3): 669–81; Kingery JE, Matheny SC. Hepatitis A. *Am Fam Physician*. 2012; 86(11): 1027–34, quiz 1010–12.

8. Caviglia GP, Abate ML, Pellicano R, Smedile A. Chronic hepatitis B therapy: Available drugs and treatment guidelines. *Minerva Gastroenterol Dietol*. 2015; 61(2): 61–70.

9. Huang CR, Lo SJ. Hepatitis D virus infection, replication and cross-talk with the hepatitis B virus. *World J Gastroenterol*. 2014; 20(40): 14589–97.

10. Irving G, Ott JJ, Wiersma ST. Long-term protective effects of hepatitis A vaccines: A systematic review. *Vaccine*. 2012; 31(1): 3–11.

11. Kohli A, Kottilil S, Shaffer A, Sherman A. Treatment of hepatitis C: A systematic review. *JAMA*. 2014; 312(6): 631–40.

12. Kmush BL, Labrique AB, Nelson KE. Risk factors for hepatitis E virus infection and disease. *Expert Rev Anti Infect Ther*. 2015; 13(1): 41–53.

13. Wagensberg J. On the existence and uniqueness of the scientific method. *Biol Theory*. 2014; 9(3): 331–46.

7. GLOBAL SCALE OF HEPATITIS

1. Abernethy NF, Au AP, Carroll LN, Detwiler LT, Fu TC, Painter IS. Visualization and analytics tools for infectious disease epidemiology: A systematic review. *J Biomed Inform*. 2014; 51: 287–98.

2. Forbi JC, Goncalves Rossi LM, Khudyakov YE, et al. Hepatitis A virus: Host interactions, molecular epidemiology and evolution. *Infect Genet Evol*. 2014; 21: 227–43.

3. Anderson BL, Hardy EJ. Communicable diseases. *Semin Reprod Med*. 2015; 33(1): 30–34.

4. Kawachi I, Koenen KC, Nishi A, Nishihara R, Ogino S, Wu K. Lifecourse epidemiology and molecular pathological epidemiology. *Am J Prev Med*. 2015; 48(1): 116–19.

5. Gluckman PD, Hanson MA. Developmental origins of health and disease: Global public health implications. *Best Pract Res Clin Obstet Gynaecol*. 2015; 29(1): 24–31.

6. Brown RS Jr, Jacobson IM, Kwo PY, Poordad F, Reddy KR, Schiff E. Standardization of terminology of virological response in the treatment of

chronic hepatitis C. Panel recommendations. *J Viral Hepat*. 2012; 19(4): 236–43.

7. Simmonds P. The origin of hepatitis C virus. *Curr Top Microbiol Immunol*. 2013; 369: 1–15.

8. Kingery JE, Matheny SC. Hepatitis A. *Am Fam Physician*. 2012; 86(11): 1027–34, quiz 1010–12; Alqahtani SA, Dhingra A, Kapoor S. Recent advances in the treatment of hepatitis C. *Discov Med*. 2014; 18(99): 203–8.

9. Wright R. Type B hepatitis: Progression to chronic hepatitis. *Clin Gastroenterol*. 1980; 9(1): 97–115.

10. Mravčík V, Reimer J, Schulte B, Strada L. Hepatitis C treatment uptake and adherence among injecting drug users in the Czech Republic. *Epidemiol Mikrobiol Imunol*. 2014; 63(4): 265–69; Ciancio A, Rizzetto M. Epidemiology of hepatitis D. *Semin Liver Dis*. 2012; 32(3): 211–19; Abravanel F, Dalton HR, Izopet J, Kamar N. Hepatitis E virus infection. *Clin Microbiol Rev*. 2014; 27(1): 116–38.

11. Holmberg SD, Jiles RB, Klevens RM, Ly KN, Xing J. Causes of death and characteristics of decedents with viral hepatitis, United States, 2010. *Clin Infect Dis*. 2014; 58(1): 40–49.

12. So AD, Ruiz-Esparza Q. Technology innovation for infectious diseases in the developing world. *Infect Dis Poverty*. 2012; 1(1): 2.

8. PATHOLOGY OF HEPATITIS

1. Procop GW, Wilson M. Infectious disease pathology. *Clin Infect Dis*. 2001; 32(11): 1589–601.

2. Guarner J. Incorporating pathology in the practice of infectious disease: Myths and reality. *Clin Infect Dis*. 2014; 59(8): 1133–41.

3. Fiel MI. Pathology of chronic hepatitis B and chronic hepatitis C. *Clin Liver Dis*. 2010; 14(4): 555–75.

4. Vajnar J. Abdominal pain in a man with hepatitis C. *JAAPA*. 2007; 20(10): 54, 57.

5. Podymova SD. Acute hepatitis in infectious diseases. *Eksp Klin Gastroenterol*. 2013; (4): 38–43.

6. Peters RL. Viral hepatitis: A pathologic spectrum. *Am J Med Sci*. 1975; 270(1): 17–31.

7. Jinjuvadia R, Lohia P, May E. Profound jaundice in a patient with acute hepatitis C. *BMJ Case Rep*. 2013; 2013; Rabson SM. Jaundice and hepatitis: A laboratory review. *Am J Dig Dis*. 1948; 15(1): 7–10.

8. Scheuer PJ. Chronic hepatitis: A problem for the pathologist. *Histopathology*. 1977; 1(1): 5–19.

9. Ferrell L. Liver pathology: Cirrhosis, hepatitis, and primary liver tumors: Update and diagnostic problems. *Mod Pathol*. 2000; 13(6): 679–704.

10. Cuthbert JA. Hepatitis A: Old and new. *Clin Microbiol Rev*. 2001; 14(1): 38–58; Liang TJ. Hepatitis B: The virus and disease. *Hepatology*. 2009; 49(5 Suppl): S13–21; Lauer GM, Walker BD. Hepatitis C virus infection. *N Engl J Med*. 2001; 345(1): 41–52; Panda SK, Thakral D, Rehman S. Hepatitis E virus. *Rev Med Virol*. 2007; 17(3): 151–80.

11. Demicheli V, Tiberti D. The effectiveness and safety of hepatitis A vaccine: A systematic review. *Vaccine*. 2003; 21(19–20): 2242–45.

12. Castera L, Constant A, Bernard PH, de Ledinghen V, Couzigou P. Lifestyle changes and beliefs regarding disease severity in patients with chronic hepatitis C. *J Viral Hepat*. 2006; 13(7): 482–88.

13. Dienstag JL, Friedman LS. Recent developments in viral hepatitis. *Dis Mon*. 1986; 32(6): 313–85; Bonkovsky HL, Ghaziani T, Sendi H, Shahraz S, Zamor P. Hepatitis B and liver transplantation: Molecular and clinical features that influence recurrence and outcome. *World J Gastroenterol*. 2014; 20(39): 14142–55.

14. Popper H. The pathology of viral hepatitis. *Can Med Assoc J*. 1972; 106(Suppl): 447–52.

9. RISK FACTORS AND CAUSES

1. Hardwick C. Hepatitis. *Guys Hosp Gaz*. 1947; 61(1530): 71–75.

2. Lowe J. An address on the germ theory of disease. *Br Med J*. 1883; 2(1176): 53–57; Katona J, Győry H, Blázovics A. Ancient medical treatments for liver disease. *Orv Hetil*. 2016; 157(48): 1926–33.

3. Glomset DA. Acute hepatitis. *J Iowa State Med Soc*. 1947; 37(3): 107–14.

4. McKell WM Jr., Mora LO. Acute alcoholic hepatitis: A review of 32 cases. *J Miss State Med Assoc*. 1970; 11(9): 477–84.

5. Larrey D, Pessayre D. Acute and chronic drug-induced hepatitis. *Baillieres Clin Gastroenterol*. 1988; 2(2): 385–422.

6. Bril F, Cusi K, Lomonaco R, Sunny NE. Nonalcoholic fatty liver disease: Current issues and novel treatment approaches. *Drugs*. 2013; 73(1): 1–14.

7. Avellón A, Echevarría JM. Hepatitis B virus genetic diversity. *J Med Virol*. 2006; 78(Suppl 1): S36–42.

8. Kato N. Genome of human hepatitis C virus (HCV): Gene organization, sequence diversity, and variation. *Microb Comp Genomics*. 2000; 5(3): 129–51.

9. Melnick JL. History and epidemiology of hepatitis A virus. *J Infect Dis*. 1995; 171(Suppl 1): S2–8.

10. Demicheli V, Tiberti D. The effectiveness and safety of hepatitis A vaccine: A systematic review. *Vaccine*. 2003; 21(19–20): 2242–45.

11. Liang TJ. Hepatitis B: The virus and disease. *Hepatology*. 2009; 49(5 Suppl): S13–21.

12. Lavanchy D. Evolving epidemiology of hepatitis C virus. *Clin Microbiol Infect*. 2011; 17(2): 107–15.

13. Taylor JM. Hepatitis delta virus. *Virology*. 2006; 344(1): 71–76.

14. Bonino F, Brunetto MR, Negro F, Ponzetto A, Smedile A. Hepatitis delta virus, a model of liver cell pathology. *J Hepatol*. 1991; 13(2): 260–66.

15. Dagan R, Jacobs RJ, Lieberman JM, Marchant CD, Word BM. Universal hepatitis A vaccination in the United States: A call for action. *Pediatr Infect Dis J*. 2008; 27(4): 287–91.

10. DIAGNOSIS OF HEPATITIS

1. Déný P, Zoulim F. Hepatitis B virus: From diagnosis to treatment. *Pathol Biol (Paris)*. 2010; 58(4): 245–53.

2. Afdhal NH. The natural history of hepatitis C. *Semin Liver Dis*. 2004; 24(Suppl 2): 3–8.

3. Collier MG, Tong X, Xu F. Hepatitis A hospitalizations in the United States, 2002–2011. *Hepatology*. 2015; 61(2): 481–85.

4. Bajpai M, Choudhary A, Gupta E. Hepatitis C virus: Screening, diagnosis, and interpretation of laboratory assays. *Asian J Transfus Sci*. 2014; 8(1): 19–25.

5. Barter DM, Horberg M, Hu H, Linas BP. Hepatitis C screening trends in a large integrated health system. *Am J Med*. 2014; 127(5): 398–405.

6. Gretch DR. Diagnostic tests for hepatitis C. *Hepatology*. 1997; 26(3 Suppl 1): 43S–47S.

7. Reuman PD, Russell BA, Sherertz RJ. Transmission of hepatits A by transfusion of blood products. *Arch Intern Med*. 1984; 144(8): 1579–80.

8. Reuman PD, Russell BA, Sherertz RJ. Transmission of hepatits A by transfusion of blood products. *Arch Intern Med*. 1984; 144(8): 1579–80.

9. Hewlett AT, Lau DT. Screening for hepatitis A and B antibodies in patients with chronic liver disease. *Am J Med*. 2005; 118(Suppl 10A): 28S–33S.

10. Boursier J, Bacq Y, Halfon P, et al. Improved diagnostic accuracy of blood tests for severe fibrosis and cirrhosis in chronic hepatitis C. *Eur J Gastroenterol Hepatol*. 2009; 21(1): 28–38.

11. Aach RD, Edwards V, Hollinger FB, et al. Hepatitis B virus antibody in blood donors and the occurrence of non-A, non-B hepatitis in transfusion recipients: An analysis of the Transfusion-Transmitted Viruses Study. *Ann Intern Med*. 1984; 101(6): 733–38.

12. Cheung RC, Keeffe EB, Yu AS. Hepatitis B vaccines. *Clin Liver Dis*. 2004; 8(2): 283–300.

13. Bacon BR, Bisceglie AM, Long GS. Interpreting serologic tests for hepatitis C virus infection: Balancing cost and clarity. *Cleve Clin J Med*. 1996; 63(5): 264–68; Aggarwal R, Jameel S. Hepatitis E. *Hepatology*. 2011; 54(6): 2218–26.

14. Caredda F, Antinori S, Pastecchia C, et al. A possible misdiagnosis in patients presenting with acute HBsAg-negative hepatitis: the role of hepatitis delta virus. *Infection*. 1988;16(6):358–9.

11. ROLE OF PRIMARY CARE PHYSICIANS

1. Dény P, Zoulim F. Hepatitis B virus: From diagnosis to treatment. *Pathol Biol (Paris)*. 2010; 58(4): 245–53.

2. Carle AC, Erikson CE, Danish S, Jones KC, Sandberg SF. The role of medical school culture in primary care career choice. *Acad Med*. 2013; 88(12): 1919–26.

3. Reede JY. Predictors of success in medicine. *Clin Orthop Relat Res*. 1999; (362): 72–77.

4. Perkowski LC, Searle NS, Thompson BM. Making it work: The evolution of a medical educational fellowship program. *Acad Med*. 2006; 81(11): 984–89.

5. Fryer GE Jr, Starfield B. The primary care physician workforce: Ethical and policy implications. *Ann Fam Med*. 2007; 5(6): 486–91; Dugdale DC, Epstein R, Pantilat SZ. Time and the patient–physician relationship. *J Gen Intern Med*. 1999; 14(Suppl 1): S34–40.

6. Burge SK, Parchman ML. The patient–physician relationship, primary care attributes, and preventive services. *Fam Med*. 2004; 36(1): 22–27.

7. Noskin GA. Prevention, diagnosis, and management of viral hepatitis: A guide for primary care physicians. AMA Advisory Group on Prevention, Diagnosis, and Management of Viral Hepatitis. *Arch Fam Med*. 1995; 4(11): 923–34.

8. Cheah SL, Tan NC. What barriers do primary care physicians face in the management of patients with chronic hepatitis B infection in primary care? *Singapore Med J*. 2005; 46(7): 333–39.

9. Lok AS, Shehab TM, Sonnad SS. Management of hepatitis C patients by primary care physicians in the USA: Results of a national survey. *J Viral Hepat*. 2001; 8(5): 377–83; Clark EC, Galliher JM, Hickner J, Temte JL, Yawn BP. Hepatitis C identification and management by family physicians. *Fam Med*. 2005; 37(9): 644–49.

10. Zevin B. Managing chronic hepatitis C in primary-care settings: More than antiviral therapy. *Public Health Rep*. 2007; 122(Suppl 2): 78–82.

12. ROLE OF HEPATOLOGISTS

1. Luxon BA. Training for a career in hepatology: Which path to take? *Curr Gastroenterol Rep*. 2010; 12(1): 76–81.

2. Bacon BR. Training in hepatology: Where are we now? *Gastroenterology*. 2009; 137(5): 1557–58.

3. Wright TL. Treatment of patients with hepatitis C and cirrhosis. *Hepatology*. 2002; 36(5 Suppl 1): S185–94.; Brown TA, Hoofnagle JH, Rotman Y. Evaluation of the patient with hepatitis B. *Hepatology*. 2009; 49(5 Suppl): S22–27.

4. Simpson SJ, Raubenheimer D, Cogger VC, et al. The nutritional geometry of liver disease including non-alcoholic fatty liver disease. *J Hepatol*. 2018; 68(2): 316–25.

5. Koff RS. Clinical manifestations and diagnosis of hepatitis A virus infection. *Vaccine*. 1992; 10 (Suppl 1): S15–17.

6. Aspinall EJ, Fraser A, Goldberg D, Hawkins G, Hutchinson SJ. Hepatitis B prevention, diagnosis, treatment and care: A review. *Occup Med (Lond)*. 2011; 61(8): 531–40.

7. Chu CJ, Lee SD. Hepatitis B virus/hepatitis C virus coinfection: Epidemiology, clinical features, viral interactions and treatment. *J Gastroenterol Hepatol*. 2008; 23(4): 512–20.

8. Lauer GM, Walker BD. Hepatitis C virus infection. *N Engl J Med*. 2001; 345(1): 41–52.

9. Perrillo RP. The role of liver biopsy in hepatitis C. *Hepatology*. 1997; 26(3 Suppl 1): 57S–61S; Jensen DM, Martin P. Ribavirin in the treatment of chronic hepatitis C. *J Gastroenterol Hepatol*. 2008; 23(6): 844–55.

10. Mishra L. The 21st century hematologist and a systems biology based approach to liver diseases. *Hepatology*. 2008; 48(6): 1731–33.

11. Nobili V, Carter-Kent C, Feldstein AE. The role of lifestyle changes in the management of chronic liver disease. *BMC Med*. 2011; 9: 70.

13. ROLE OF GASTROENTEROLOGISTS

1. Dienstag JL, McHutchison JG. American Gastroenterological Association technical review on the management of hepatitis C. *Gastroenterology*. 2006; 130(1): 231–64, quiz 214–17.

2. Barton R, Inglis S, Wells CW. Trainees in gastroenterology views on teaching in clinical gastroenterology and endoscopy. *Med Teach*. 2009; 31(2): 138–44.

3. Law R, Singla MB. Gastroenterology fellowship programs: The fellows' perspective. *Clin Transl Gastroenterol*. 2015; 6: e83.

4. Czaja AJ, Manns MP. Advances in the diagnosis, pathogenesis, and management of autoimmune hepatitis. *Gastroenterology*. 2010; 139(1): 58–72e4.

5. Grace ND, Reddy SI. Liver imaging: A hepatologist's perspective. *Clin Liver Dis*. 2002; 6(1): 297–310, ix.

6. Huffman MM, Mounsey AL. Hepatitis C for primary care physicians. *J Am Board Fam Med*. 2014; 27(2): 284–91.

7. Dienstag JL, McHutchison JG. American Gastroenterological Association medical position statement on the management of hepatitis C. *Gastroenterology*. 2006; 130(1): 225–30.

8. Beyazit Y, Guclu M, Gulsen MT, Koklu S. Testing for hepatitis B and C virus infection before upper gastrointestinal endoscopy: Justification for dedicated endoscope and room for hepatitis patients. *Hepatogastroenterology*. 2010; 57(101): 797–800.

9. Almario CV, Navarro VJ, Trooskin SB, Vega M. Examining hepatitis C virus testing practices in primary care clinics. *J Viral Hepat*. 2012; 19(2): e163–69.

10. Comanor L, Holland P. Hepatitis B virus blood screening: Unfinished agendas. *Vox Sang*. 2006; 91(1): 1–12.

11. Dubé C. Tackling colorectal cancer as a public health issue: What can the gastroenterologist do? *Can J Gastroenterol*. 2012; 26(7): 417–18.

14. ROLE OF HOSPITALS

1. Anderson RJ, Boumbulian PJ, Pickens SS. The role of U.S. public hospitals in urban health. *Acad Med*. 2004; 79(12): 1162–68.

2. Dopson S, Parand A, Renz A, Vincent C. The role of hospital managers in quality and patient safety: A systematic review. *BMJ Open*. 2014; 4(9): e005055.

3. Chatterjee A, Dutta S, Shivananda PG. Prevalence of hepatitis B surface antigen and antibody among hospital admitted patients in Manipal. *Indian J Public Health*. 1994; 38(3): 108–12; Antony J, Celine T. A hospital-based retrospective study on frequency and distribution of viral hepatitis. *J Glob Infect Dis*. 2014; 6(3): 99–104.

4. Elizee PK, Alavian SM. Prevention of hepatitis a virus infection, need to vaccinate or not? *Int J Prev Med*. 2013; 4(8): 863–65.

5. Hierholzer WR, LaBrecque DR, Lutwick LI, Muhs JM, Woolson RF. The risk of hepatitis B transmission from health care workers to patients in a hospital setting: A prospective study. *Hepatology*. 1986; 6(2): 205–8; Fukushima Y, Ishikawa T, Kishimoto T, et al. Outbreak of hepatitis C virus infection in an outpatient clinic. *J Gastroenterol Hepatol*. 2005; 20(7): 1087–93; Edmond MB, Wenzel RP. Patient-to-patient transmission of hepatitis C virus. *Ann Intern Med*. 2005; 142(11): 940–41; Arsalla Z, Henry L, Hunt S, et al. Inpatient resource utilization, disease severity, mortality and insurance coverage for patients hospitalized for hepatitis C virus in the United States. *J Viral Hepat*. 2015; 22(2): 137–45.

6. Dixon RE, Favero MS, Graham DR, Leger RT, Maynard JE. Guidelines for the care of patients hospitalized with viral hepatitis. *Ann Intern Med*. 1979; 91(6): 872–76; Berthelot P, Garraud O, Memmi M, Ozzetto B, Roblin X. Health care-associated hepatitis C virus infection. *World J Gastroenterol*. 2014; 20(46): 17265–78.

7. Chung RT, Feeney ER. Antiviral treatment of hepatitis C. *BMJ*. 2014; 348: g3308.

8. Cornberg M, Manns MP, Wedemeyer H. Treating viral hepatitis C: Efficacy, side effects, and complications. *Gut*. 2006; 55(9): 1350–59.

9. Cupane L, Dumpis U, Gardovska D, et al. An outbreak of HBV and HCV infection in a paediatric oncology ward: Epidemiological investigations and prevention of further spread. *J Med Virol*. 2003; 69(3): 331–38.

10. Ho SB. What defines high quality care for patients with chronic hepatitis C and why should we care? *Dig Dis Sci*. 2014; 59(2): 233–34.

15. HEPATITIS AND CHOLESTEROL

1. Ghadir MR, Riahin AA, Havaspour A, et al. The relationship between lipid profile and severity of liver damage in cirrhotic patients. *Hepat Mon*. 2010; 10(4): 285–88.

2. Koudinov AR, Koudinova NV. Cholesterol, synaptic function and Alzheimer's disease. *Pharmacopsychiatry*. 2003; 36(Suppl 2): S107–12.

3. Siri-Tarino PW. Effects of diet on high-density lipoprotein cholesterol. *Curr Atheroscler Rep*. 2011; 13(6): 453–60.

4. Eaton CB. Hyperlipidemia. *Prim Care*. 2005; 32(4): 1027–55, viii.

5. Avins AL, Hulley SB. Screening for high cholesterol. *J Gen Intern Med*. 1990; 5(1): 88–89.

6. Criqui MH. Cholesterol, primary and secondary prevention, and all-cause mortality. *Ann Intern Med*. 1991; 115(12): 973–76.

7. Chan KS, Hebert PR, Hennekens CH, Gaziano JM. Cholesterol lowering with statin drugs, risk of stroke, and total mortality: An overview of randomized trials. *JAMA*. 1997; 278(4): 313–21.

8. Doy M, Hara T, Hirayama T, et al. Hepatitis C virus infection causes hypolipidemia regardless of hepatic damage or nutritional state: An epidemiological survey of a large Japanese cohort. *Hepatol Res*. 2011; 41(6): 530–41; Chen CH, Chuang TW, Hu TH, et al. Reversal of hypolipidemia in chronic hepatitis C patients after successful antiviral therapy. *J Formos Med Assoc*. 2011; 110(6): 363–71.

9. Chang MH. Prevention of hepatitis B virus infection and liver cancer. *Recent Results Cancer Res*. 2014; 193: 75–95.

10. Akhan SC, Gurel E, Sayan M. The sustained virologic response of nonresponder hepatitis C virus patients with pretreatment. *Indian J Pathol Microbiol*. 2011; 54(1): 81–84; Cerri K, Smith-Palmer J, Valentine W. Achieving sustained virologic response in hepatitis C: A systematic review of the clinical, economic and quality of life benefits. *BMC Infect Dis*. 2015; 15: 19.

11. Aston C, Bader T, Fazili J, et al. Fluvastatin inhibits hepatitis C replication in humans. *Am J Gastroenterol*. 2008; 103(6): 1383–89.

16. HEPATITIS AND OBESITY

1. Haslam DW, James WP. *Obesity. Lancet*. 2005; 366(9492): 1197–209.

2. Bray GA. Risks of obesity. *Endocrinol Metab Clin North Am*. 2003; 32(4): 787–804, viii; Pi-Sunyer X. The medical risks of obesity. *Postgrad Med*. 2009; 121(6): 21–33.

3. Honda A, Matsuzaki Y. Cholesterol and chronic hepatitis C virus infection. *Hepatol Res*. 2011; 41(8): 697–710.

4. Basaranoglu M, Basaranoglu G, Bugianesi E. Carbohydrate intake and nonalcoholic fatty liver disease: Fructose as a weapon of mass destruction. *Hepatobiliary Surg Nutr*. 2015; 4(2): 109–16.

5. Goran MI. Energy metabolism and obesity. *Med Clin North Am*. 2000; 84(2): 347–62; Ruhm CJ. Understanding overeating and obesity. *J Health Econ*. 2012; 31(6): 781–96.

6. Fernstrom MH. Drugs that cause weight gain. *Obes Res*. 1995; 3(Suppl 4): 435S–39.

7. Fernstrom MH. Drugs that cause weight gain. *Obes Res*. 1995; 3(Suppl 4): 435S–39S.

8. Minihane AM, Vinoy S, Russell WR, et al. Low-grade inflammation, diet composition and health: Current research evidence and its translation. *Br J Nutr*. 2015; 114(7): 999–1012.

9. Bensimhon DR, Donahue MP, Kraus WE. Obesity and physical activity: A review. *Am Heart J*. 2006; 151(3): 598–603; Isaac R, Jacob JJ. Behavioral therapy for management of obesity. *Indian J Endocrinol Metab*. 2012; 16(1): 28–32.

10. Uusitupa M. New aspects in the management of obesity: Operation and the impact of lipase inhibitors. *Curr Opin Lipidol*. 1999; 10(1): 3–7.

11. Flier JS, Kahn BB. Obesity and insulin resistance. *J Clin Invest*. 2000; 106(4): 473–81; Seeff LB. Sustained virologic response: Is this equivalent to cure of chronic hepatitis C? *Hepatology*. 2013; 57(2): 438–40.

12. Charlton MR, Harrison SA, Pockros PJ. Impact of obesity on treatment of chronic hepatitis C. *Hepatology*. 2006; 43(6): 1177–86; Poynard T, Ratziu V, Trabut JB. Fat, diabetes, and liver injury in chronic hepatitis C. *Curr Gastroenterol Rep*. 2004; 6(1): 22–29.

17. HEPATITIS AND HEART DISEASE

1. Matsumori A. Hepatitis C virus infection and cardiomyopathies. *Circ Res*. 2005; 96(2): 144–47.

2. Lusis AJ. Atherosclerosis. *Nature*. 2000; 407(6801): 233–41; Adams MJ, Block RC, Cohn SE, Fisher SG, Kakinami L, Maliakkal B. Risk of cardiovascular disease in HIV, hepatitis C, or HIV/hepatitis C patients compared to the general population. *Int J Clin Pract*. 2013; 67(1): 6–13.

3. Chen TL, Chou WH, Liao CC, Su TC, Sung FC. Does hepatitis C virus infection increase risk for stroke? A population-based cohort study. *PLoS One*. 2012; 7(2): e31527.

4. Elsheikh E, Nader F, Stepanova M, Younossi ZM, Younossi Z. Associations of chronic hepatitis C with metabolic and cardiac outcomes. *Aliment Pharmacol Ther*. 2013; 37(6): 647–52.

5. Demir C, Demir M. Effect of hepatitis B virus infection on right and left ventricular functions. *Med Sci Monit*. 2012; 18(9): CR587–91.

6. Matsumori A. Hepatitis C virus infection and cardiomyopathies. *Circ Res*. 2005; 96(2): 144–47.

7. Kjaer A, Lebech AM, Roed T, Weis N. Hepatitis C virus infection and risk of coronary artery disease: A systematic review of the literature. *Clin Physiol Funct Imaging*. 2012; 32(6): 421–30; Bianchi F, Vassalle C, Masini S, Zucchelli GC. Evidence for association between hepatitis C virus seropositivity and coronary artery disease. *Heart*. 2004; 90(5): 565–66.

8. Matsumori A. Hepatitis C virus infection and cardiomyopathies. *Circ Res*. 2005; 96(2): 144–47.

9. Mangi MA, Minhas AM, Rehman H, Pathan F, Liang H, Beidas S. Association of non-alcoholic fatty liver disease with conduction defects on electrocardiogram. *Cureus*. 2017; 9(3): e1107.

10. Gillum RF. Diagnostic technology in cardiovascular disease: Review of noninvasive methods for population studies. *Bull World Health Organ*. 1988; 66(2): 249–58; Gupta AK, Kapoor KK, Kumar A, Nigam P. Electrocardiographic changes in acute viral hepatitis. *J Assoc Physicians India*. 1986; 34(12): 841–43.

11. Perez-Terzic CM. Exercise in cardiovascular diseases. *PM&R*. 2012; 4(11): 867–73.

12. Chapman NM, Mason JW, Matsumori A, Shimada T, Tracy SM. Myocarditis and heart failure associated with hepatitis C virus infection. *J Card Fail*. 2006; 12(4): 293–98.

13. Matsumori A. Hepatitis C virus and cardiomyopathy. *Herz*. 2000; 25(3): 249–54.

18. HEPATITIS AND LIVER CANCER

1. Ringelhan M, McKeating JA, Protzer U. Viral hepatitis and liver cancer. *Philos Trans R Soc Lond B Biol Sci*. 2017; 372(1732).

2. Bissell MJ, Radisky D. Putting tumors in context. *Nat Rev Cancer*. 2001; 1(1): 46–54; Carmeliet P, Jain RK. Angiogenesis in cancer and other diseases. *Nature*. 2000; 407(6801): 249–57.

3. Bloomfield CD, Caligiuri MA, Coller H, et al. Molecular classification of cancer: Class discovery and class prediction by gene expression monitoring. *Science*. 1999; 286(5439): 531–37.

4. Chang MH. Hepatitis B virus and cancer prevention. *Recent Results Cancer Res*. 2011; 188: 75–84.

5. Chang MH. Prevention of hepatitis B virus infection and liver cancer. *Recent Results Cancer Res*. 2014; 193: 75–95; Fattovich G, Brouwer JT, Schalm SW. Therapy of hepatitis C: Patients with cirrhosis. *Hepatology*. 1997; 26(3 Suppl 1): 128S–32S.

6. Kawarada Y, Mizumoto R. Cholangiocellular carcinoma of the liver. *Am J Surg*. 1984; 147(3): 354–59.

7. Freelove R, Walling AD. Pancreatic cancer: Diagnosis and management. *Am Fam Physician*. 2006; 73(3): 485–92.

8. Cairns RA, Harris IS, Mak TW. Regulation of cancer cell metabolism. *Nat Rev Cancer*. 2011; 11(2): 85–95.

9. Martin DR, Namasivayam S, Saini S. Imaging of liver metastases: MRI. *Cancer Imaging*. 2007; 7: 2–9.

10. Shindoh J, Hashimoto M, Watanabe G. Surgical approach for hepatitis C virus-related hepatocellular carcinoma. *World J Hepatol*. 2015; 7(1): 70–77.

11. Shindoh J, Hashimoto M, Watanabe G. Surgical approach for hepatitis C virus-related hepatocellular carcinoma. *World J Hepatol*. 2015; 7(1): 70–77.

12. McCarley JR, Soulen MC. Percutaneous ablation of hepatic tumors. *Semin Intervent Radiol*. 2010; 27(3): 255–60.

13. Chang MH. Cancer prevention by vaccination against hepatitis B. *Recent Results Cancer Res*. 2009; 181: 85–94.

14. Alter MJ. Epidemiology and prevention of hepatitis B. *Semin Liver Dis*. 2003; 23(1): 39–46; Ozaras R, Tahan V. Acute hepatitis C: Prevention and treatment. *Expert Rev Anti Infect Ther*. 2009; 7(3): 351–61.

15. Armstrong GL, Bell BP, Farrington LA, Hutin YJ, Perz JF. The contributions of hepatitis B virus and hepatitis C virus infections to cirrhosis and primary liver cancer worldwide. *J Hepatol*. 2006; 45(4): 529–38; Barazani Y, Busuttil RW, Hiatt JR, Tong MJ. Chronic viral hepatitis and hepatocellular carcinoma. *World J Surg*. 2007; 31(6): 1243–48.

19. TYPES OF LIVER DISORDERS

1. Koike H, Zhang RR, Ueno Y, et al. Nutritional modulation of mouse and human liver bud growth through a branched-chain amino acid metabolism. *Development*. 2017 Mar 15;144(6):1018–1024.

2. Arguedas MR, Fallon MB. Prevention in liver disease. *Am J Med Sci*. 2001; 321(2): 145–51.

3. Brůha R, Dousa M, Dvorák K, Petrtýl J, Svestka T. Alcoholic liver disease. *Prague Med Rep*. 2009; 110(3): 181–90.

4. Mieli-Vergani G, Vergani D. Autoimmune paediatric liver disease. *World J Gastroenterol*. 2008; 14(21): 3360–67.

5. Morgan MY. The prognosis and outcome of alcoholic liver disease. *Alcohol Alcohol*. 1994; 2(Suppl): 335–43; Morgan MY. The treatment of alcoholic hepatitis. *Alcohol Alcohol*. 1996; 31(2): 117–34.

6. Donato F, Fattovich G, Stroffolini T, Zagni I. Hepatocellular carcinoma in cirrhosis: Incidence and risk factors. *Gastroenterology*. 2004; 127(5 Suppl 1): S35–50; Monto A, Wright TL. The epidemiology and prevention of hepatocellular carcinoma. *Semin Oncol*. 2001; 28(5): 441–49.

7. Reid AE. Nonalcoholic steatohepatitis. *Gastroenterology*. 2001; 121(3): 710–23.

8. Bruix J, Forner A, Llovet JM. Hepatocellular carcinoma. *Lancet*. 2012; 379(9822): 1245–55.

9. Barakat R, el-Morshedy H, Farghaly A, Sharaf S, Abou-Basha L. Triclabendazole in the treatment of human fascioliasis: A community-based study. *East Mediterr Health J*. 1999; 5(5): 888–94; Price TA, Simon GL, Tuazon CU. Fascioliasis: Case reports and review. *Clin Infect Dis*. 1993; 17(3): 426–30.

10. Powell LW, Yapp TR. Hemochromatosis. *Clin Liver Dis*. 2000; 4(1): 211–28, viii.

11. Kryczka W, Kubicka J, Lembowicz K, Walewska-Zielecka B. Wilson's disease coexisting with viral hepatitis type C: A case report with histological and ultrastructural studies of the liver. *Ultrastruct Pathol*. 1999; 23(1): 39–44.

12. Lok AS, Scaglione SJ. Effectiveness of hepatitis B treatment in clinical practice. *Gastroenterology*. 2012; 142(6): 1360–68.e1; Lok AS, Jafri SM. Antiviral therapy for chronic hepatitis B. *Clin Liver Dis*. 2010; 14(3): 425–38.

20. RELATED NONHEPATIC DISORDERS

1. Buskila D. Hepatitis C-associated rheumatic disorders. *Rheum Dis Clin North Am*. 2009; 35(1): 111–23.

2. Bresnahan M, Link BG, Pescosolido BA, Phelan JC, Stueve A. Public conceptions of mental illness: Labels, causes, dangerousness, and social distance. *Am J Public Health*. 1999; 89(9): 1328–33.

3. Floreani A. Hepatitis C and pregnancy. *World J Gastroenterol*. 2013; 19(40): 6714–20.

4. Davis RB, Iezzoni LI, McCarthy EP, Siebens H. Mobility impairments and use of screening and preventive services. *Am J Public Health*. 2000; 90(6): 955–61; Fried LP, Prasada-Rao P, Roche KB, Rubin GS. Visual impairment and disability in older adults. *Optom Vis Sci*. 1994; 71(12): 750–60.

5. Busse WW, Lemanske RF Jr. Asthma. *N Engl J Med*. 2001; 344(5): 350–62.

6. Collins MM, Corcoran P, Perry IJ. Anxiety and depression symptoms in patients with diabetes. *Diabet Med*. 2009; 26(2): 153–61.

7. Innes E, Van Huet H, Whiteford G. Living and doing with chronic pain: Narratives of pain program participants. *Disabil Rehabil.* 2009; 31(24): 2031–40.

8. Bell EJ, Dowsett EG, McCartney RA, Ramsay AM. Myalgic encephalomyelitis: A persistent enteroviral infection? *Postgrad Med J.* 1990; 66(777): 526–30.

9. Cam S, Ertem D, Koroglu OA, Pehlivanoglu E. Hepatitis A virus infection presenting with seizures. *Pediatr Infect Dis J.* 2005; 24(7): 652–53.

10. Miles JH. Autism spectrum disorders: A genetics review. *Genet Med.* 2011; 13(4): 278–94.

11. Miyahara M, Möbs I. Developmental dyspraxia and developmental coordination disorder. *Neuropsychol Rev.* 1995; 5(4): 245–68.

12. Leung N. Treatment of chronic hepatitis B: Case selection and duration of therapy. J *Gastroenterol Hepatol.* 2002; 17(4): 409–14.

21. NATURAL APPROACHES FOR HEPATITIS

1. Niggemann B1, Grüber C. Side-effects of complementary and alternative medicine. *Allergy.* 2003; 58(8): 707–16.

2. Lin H, Liu JP, McIntosh H. Chinese medicinal herbs for chronic hepatitis B. *Cochrane Database Syst Rev.* 2001; (1): CD001940.

3. Coon JT, Ernst E. Complementary and alternative therapies in the treatment of chronic hepatitis C: A systematic review. *J Hepatol.* 2004; 40(3): 491–500.

4. Chen X, Lu Y, Xu Q, Yang Z, Zhuang L. Effects and tolerance of silymarin (milk thistle) in chronic hepatitis C virus infection patients: A meta-analysis of randomized controlled trials. *Biomed Res Int.* 2014; 2014: 941085.

5. Ashfaq UA, Masoud MS, Nawaz Z, Riazuddin S. Glycyrrhizin as antiviral agent against hepatitis C virus. *J Transl Med.* 2011; 9: 112.

6. Caredda F, Crocchiolo P, Galli M, Lazzarin A, Moroni M, Negri C. Attempt to treat acute type B hepatitis with an orally administered thymic extract (thymomodulin): Preliminary results. *Drugs Exp Clin Res.* 1985; 11(9): 665–69.

7. Cui X, Fang D, Kokudo N, Tang W, Wang Y. Traditional Chinese medicine and related active compounds against hepatitis B virus infection. *Biosci Trends.* 2010; 4(2): 39–47.

8. Correia MI, Menta PL, Silva LD, Teixeira R, Vidigal PV. Nutrition status of patients with chronic hepatitis B or C. *Nutr Clin Pract.* 2015; 30(2): 290–96; Kaur H, Singh P, Pannu HS, Sood A, Jain NP, Bhoday HS. To study

the prevalence of impaired glucose tolerance in patients with hepatitis C virus related chronic liver disease. *J Clin Diagn Res*. 2015; 9(3): OC16–20.

9. Soffer A. Editorial: Chicken soup, sippy milk diets and bed rest for hepatitis. *Chest*. 1975; 67(2): 214–15.

10. Hammerstad SS, Grock SF, Lee HJ et al. Diabetes and hepatitis c: A two-way association. *Front Endocrinal*. 2015 Sep 14; 6:134.

11. Ateia S, Ancuta I, Cheţa DM, et al. Effects of lifestyle changes including specific dietary intervention and physical activity in the management of patients with chronic hepatitis C: A randomized trial. *Nutr J*. 2013; 12: 119; Li G, Li H, Song J, Qin H, Wu C, Xing M. Nutritional support treatment for severe chronic hepatitis and posthepatitic cirrhosis. *J Huazhong Univ Sci Technolog Med Sci*. 2006; 26(2): 217–20.

12. Denniston MM, Jiles RB, Drobeniuc J, et al. Chronic hepatitis C virus infection in the United States, national health and nutrition examination survey 2003 to 2010. *Ann Intern Med*. 2014; 160(5): 293–300; Antar R, Wong P, Ghali P. A meta analysis of nutritional supplementation for management of hospitalized alcoholic hepatitis. *Can J Gastroenterol*. 2012; 26(7): 463–67; Andreone P, Fiorino S, Cursaro C, et al. Vitamin E as treatment for chronic hepatitis B: Results of a randomized controlled pilot trial. *Antiviral Res*. 2001; 49(2): 75–81; Fiorino S, Conti F, Gramenzi A, et al. Vitamins in the treatment of chronic viral hepatitis. *Br J Nutr*. 2011; 105(7): 982–89.

13. Azzam HS, Goertz C, Fritts M, Jonas WB. Natural products and chronic hepatitis C virus. *Liver Int*. 2007; 27(1): 17–25.

22. EXERCISE FOR HEPATITIS PATIENTS

1. Harrington DW. Viral hepatitis and exercise. *Med Sci Sports Exerc*. 2000; 32(7 Suppl): S422–30.

2. Berryman JW. Exercise is medicine: A historical perspective. *Curr Sports Med Rep*. 2010; 9(4): 195–201; Mondal S. Science of exercise: Ancient Indian origin. *J Assoc Physicians India*. 2013; 61(8): 560–62.

3. Kleisiaris CF, Papathanasiou IV, Sfakianakis C. Health care practices in ancient Greece: The Hippocratic ideal. *J Med Ethics Hist Med*. 2014; 7: 6.

4. Ross A, Thomas S. The health benefits of yoga and exercise: A review of comparison studies. *J Altern Complement Med*. 2010; 16(1): 3–12.

5. Harrington DW. Viral hepatitis and exercise. *Med Sci Sports Exerc*. 2000; 32(7 Suppl): S422–30.

6. Shida A, Sumiya N, Ueno F. The effects of physical activity on rehabilitation for acute hepatitis. *Tokai J Exp Clin Med*. 1996; 21(1): 1–6; Gloth MJ,

Matesi AM. Physical therapy and exercise in pain management. *Clin Geriatr Med*. 2001; 17(3): 525–35, vii.

7. Johnson NA, Keating SE, George J. Exercise and the liver: Implications for therapy in fatty liver disorders. *Semin Liver Dis*. 2012; 32(1): 65–79. Chen CJ, Lin CL, Liu CJ, et al. Body-mass index and progression of hepatitis B: A population-based cohort study in men. *J Clin Oncol*. 2008; 26(34): 5576–82; Heathcote J. Weighty issues in hepatitis C. *Gut*. 2002; 51(1): 7–8.

8. Bridden C, Cheng DM, Libman H, Samet J, Tsui JI. Hepatitis C virus infection is associated with painful symptoms in HIV-infected adults. *AIDS Care*. 2012; 24(7): 820–27; Koerbel LS, Zucker DM. The suitability of mindfulness-based stress reduction for chronic hepatitis C. *Holist Nurs*. 2007; 25(4): 265–74; quiz, 275–77.

9. Bridden C, Cheng DM, Libman H, Samet J, Tsui JI. Hepatitis C virus infection is associated with painful symptoms in HIV-infected adults. *AIDS Care*. 2012; 24(7): 820–27; Koerbel LS, Zucker DM. The suitability of mindfulness-based stress reduction for chronic hepatitis C. *Holist Nurs*. 2007; 25(4): 265–74; quiz, 275–77.

10. Shephard RJ, Johnson N. Effects of physical activity upon the liver. *Eur J Appl Physiol*. 2015; 115(1): 1–46; Brolinson PG, Elliott D. Exercise and the immune system. *Clin Sports Med*. 2007; 26(3): 311–19.

23. PHARMACOLOGICAL APPROACHES TO HEPATITIS

1. Lagaye S, Brun S, Gaston J, et al. Anti-hepatitis C virus potency of a new autophagy inhibitor using human liver slices model. *World J Hepatol*. 2016; 8(21): 902–14.

2. Kelly DA. Managing liver failure. *Postgrad Med J*. 2002; 78(925): 660–67; Kjaer D, Horvath-Puhó E, Christensen J, et al. Use of phenytoin, phenobarbital, or diazepam during pregnancy and risk of congenital abnormalities: A case-time-control study. *Pharmacoepidemiol Drug Saf*. 2007; 16(2): 181–88.

3. Krause L, Shuster S. Mechanism of action of antipruritic drugs. *Br Med J (Clin Res Ed)*. 1983; 287(6400): 1199–200; Hofstee HM, Nanayakkara PW, Stehouwer CD. Acute hepatitis related to prednisolone. *Eur J Intern Med*. 2005; 16(3): 209–10; Buchman AL. Side effects of corticosteroid therapy. *J ClinGastroenterol*. 2001; 33(4): 289–94.

4. Soriano V, Labarga P, Fernandez-Montero JV, et al. Hepatitis C cure with antiviral therapy: Benefits beyond the liver. *Antivir Ther*. 2015.

5. Tassopoulos NC, Koutelou MG, Polychronaki H, Paraloglou-Ioannides M, Hadziyannis SJ. Recombinant interferon-alpha therapy for acute hepatitis B: A randomized, double-blind, placebo-controlled trial. *J Viral Hepat*. 1997; 4(6): 387–94.

6. Wang G, Liu Y, Qiu P, et al. Cost-effectiveness analysis of lamivudine, telbivudine, and entecavir in treatment of chronic hepatitis B with adefovirdipivoxil resistance. *Drug Des Devel Ther*. 2015; 9: 2839–46; Holland PV, Alter HJ. Non-A, non-B viral hepatitis. *Hum Pathol*. 1981; 12(12): 1114–22.

7. Stewart BJ, Mikocka-Walus AA, Harley H, Andrews JM. Help-seeking and coping with the psychosocial burden of chronic hepatitis C: A qualitative study of patient, hepatologist, and counsellor perspectives. *Int J Nurs Stud*. 2012; 49(5): 560–69; Idilman R, De Maria N, Colantoni A, Dokmeci A, Van Thiel DH. Interferon treatment of cirrhotic patients with chronic hepatitis C. *J Viral Hepat*. 1997; 4(2): 81–91; Fried MW. Side effects of therapy of hepatitis C and their management. *Hepatology*. 2002; 36(5 Suppl 1): S237–44.

8. Wilson IB, Schoen C, Neuman P, et al. Physician–patient communication about prescription medication nonadherence: A 50-state study of America's seniors. *J Gen Intern Med*. 2007; 22(1): 6–12.

24. HEPATITIS AND SURGERY

1. Fisher WD. Hepatitis C and the surgeon. *Can J Surg*. 2013; 56(2): 80–81.

2. Crespo G, Mariño Z, Navasa M, Forns X. Viral hepatitis in liver transplantation. *Gastroenterology*. 2012; 142(6): 1373–83; Morgan MY. The prognosis and outcome of alcoholic liver disease. *Alcohol Alcohol*. 1994; 2(Suppl): 335–43.

3. Kennedy M, Alexopoulos SP. Hepatitis B virus infection and liver transplantation. *Curr Opin Organ Transplant*. 2010; 15(3): 310–15; Todo S, Demetris AJ, Van Thiel D, Teperman L, Fung JJ, Starzl TE. Orthotopic liver transplantation for patients with hepatitis B virus-related liver disease. *Hepatology*. 1991; 13(4): 619–26.

4. Kennedy M, Alexopoulos SP. Hepatitis B virus infection and liver transplantation. *Curr Opin Organ Transplant*. 2010; 15(3): 310–15; Todo S, Demetris AJ, Van Thiel D, Teperman L, Fung JJ, Starzl TE. Orthotopic liver transplantation for patients with hepatitis B virus-related liver disease. *Hepatology*. 1991; 13(4): 619–26.

5. Reddy SK, Barbas AS, Turley RS, et al. A standard definition of major hepatectomy: Resection of four or more liver segments. *HPB (Oxford)*. 2011; 13(7): 494–502.

6. Alqahtani SA. Update in liver transplantation. *Curr Opin Gastroenterol*. 2012; 28(3): 230–38; Sutherland LM, Williams JA, Padbury RT, Gotley DC, Stokes B, Maddern GJ. Radiofrequency ablation of liver tumors: A systematic review. *Arch Surg*. 2006; 141(2): 181–90.

7. Tan HH, Fiel MI, del Rio MJ, Schiano TD. Graft rejection occurring in post-liver transplant patients receiving cytotoxic chemotherapy: A case series. *Liver Transpl*. 2009; 15(6): 634–39; Della-Guardia B, Almeida MD, Meira-Filho SP. Antibody-mediated rejection: Hyperacute rejection reality in liver transplantation? A case report. *Transplant Proc*. 2008; 40(3): 870–71; Wang YC, Wu TJ, Wu TH, et al. The risk factors to predict acute rejection in liver transplantation. *Transplant Proc*. 2012; 44(2): 526–28.

8. Freese DK, Snover DC, Sharp HL, Gross CR, Savick SK, Payne WD. Chronic rejection after liver transplantation: A study of clinical, histopathological and immunological features. *Hepatology*. 1991; 13(5): 882–91.

9. Nicoll A. Surgical risk in patients with cirrhosis. *J Gastroenterol Hepatol*. 2012; 27(10): 1569–75.

25. MENTAL ASPECTS

1. Manos MM, Ho CK, Murphy RC, Shvachko VA. Physical, social, and psychological consequences of treatment for hepatitis C: A community-based evaluation of patient-reported outcomes. *Patient*. 2013; 6(1): 23–34; Walter S, Leissner N, Jerg-Bretzke L, Hrabal V, Traue HC. Pain and emotional processing in psychological trauma. *Psychiatr Danub*. 2010; 22(3): 465–70; Qureshi MO, Khokhar N, Shafqat F. Severity of depression in hepatitis B and hepatitis C patients. *J Coll Physicians Surg Pak*. 2012; 22(10): 632–34.

2. Manos MM, Ho CK, Murphy RC, Shvachko VA. Physical, social, and psychological consequences of treatment for hepatitis C: A community-based evaluation of patient-reported outcomes. *Patient*. 2013; 6(1): 23–34.

3. Walter S, Leissner N, Jerg-Bretzke L, Hrabal V, Traue HC. Pain and emotional processing in psychological trauma. *Psychiatr Danub*. 2010; 22(3): 465–70; Qureshi MO, Khokhar N, Shafqat F. Severity of depression in hepatitis B and hepatitis C patients. *J Coll Physicians Surg Pak*. 2012; 22(10): 632–34.

4. Menta PL, Correia MI, Vidigal PV, Silva LD, Teixeira R. Nutrition status of patients with chronic hepatitis B or C. *Nutr Clin Pract*. 2015; 30(2): 290–96.

5. Swain MG. Fatigue in liver disease: Pathophysiology and clinical management. *Can J Gastroenterol*. 2006; 20(3): 181–88.

6. Swain MG. Fatigue in liver disease: Pathophysiology and clinical management. *Can J Gastroenterol*. 2006; 20(3): 181–88.

7. Gill ML, Atiq M, Sattar S, Khokhar N. Psychological implications of hepatitis C virus diagnosis. *J Gastroenterol Hepatol*. 2005; 20(11): 1741–44.

26. ADJUSTING TO LIFE AS A HEPATITIS PATIENT

1. Gardner B, Lally P, Wardle J. Making health habitual: The psychology of "habit-formation" and general practice. *Br J Gen Pract*. 2012; 62(605): 664–66.

2. Zandi M, Adib-Hajbagheri M, Memarian R, Nejhad AK, Alavian SM. Effects of a self-care program on quality of life of cirrhotic patients referring to Tehran Hepatitis Center. *Health Qual Life Outcomes*. 2005; 3: 35.

3. Stephensen CB. Vitamin A, infection, and immune function. *Annu Rev Nutr*. 2001; 21: 167–92.

4. Fabris P, Tositti G, Giordani MT, et al. Assessing patients' understanding of hepatitis C virus infection and its impact on their lifestyle. *Aliment Pharmacol Ther*. 2006; 23(8): 1161–70; Castera L, Constant A, Bernard PH, de Ledinghen V, Couzigou P. Lifestyle changes and beliefs regarding disease severity in patients with chronic hepatitis C. *J Viral Hepat*. 2006; 13(7): 482–88.

5. Fabris P, Tositti G, Giordani MT, et al. Assessing patients' understanding of hepatitis C virus infection and its impact on their lifestyle. *Aliment Pharmacol Ther*. 2006; 23(8): 1161–70; Castera L, Constant A, Bernard PH, de Ledinghen V, Couzigou P. Lifestyle changes and beliefs regarding disease severity in patients with chronic hepatitis C. *J Viral Hepat*. 2006; 13(7): 482–88.

6. Ramsøe K, Andreasen PB, Ranek L. Functioning liver mass in uncomplicated and fulminant acute hepatitis. *Scand J Gastroenterol*. 1980; 15(1): 65–72.

7. Malaguarnera G, Cataudella E, Giordano M, Nunnari G, Chisari G, Malaguarnera M. Toxic hepatitis in occupational exposure to solvents. *World J Gastroenterol*. 2012; 18(22): 2756–66; Caciari T, Casale T, Pimpinella B, et al. Exposure to solvents in health care workers: Assessment of the hepatic effects. *Ann Ig*. 2013; 25(2): 125–36.

8. Liang TJ. Hepatitis B: The virus and disease. *Hepatology*. 2009; 49(5 Suppl): S13–21; Lauer GM, Walker BD. Hepatitis C virus infection. *N Engl J Med*. 2001; 345(1): 41–52; Sgorbini M, O'Brien L, Jackson D. Living with

hepatitis C and treatment: The personal experiences of patients. *J Clin Nurs*. 2009; 18(16): 2282–91.

9. Geier MR, Geier DA. Hepatitis B vaccination safety. *Ann Pharmacother*. 2002; 36(3): 370–74; Geier MR, Geier DA, Zahalsky AC. A review of hepatitis B vaccination. *Expert Opin Drug Saf*. 2003; 2(2): 113–22.

10. Ockene JK, Sorensen G, Kabat-Zinn J, Ockene IS, Donnelly G. Benefits and costs of lifestyle change to reduce risk of chronic disease. *Prev Med*. 1988; 17(2): 224–34.

27. ADVANCEMENTS IN HEPATITIS RESEARCH

1. Bhatt A. Evolution of clinical research: A history before and beyond James Lind. *Perspect Clin Res*. 2010; 1(1): 6–10.

2. Kmieć Z. Cooperation of liver cells in health and disease. *Adv Anat Embryol Cell Biol*. 2001; 161: iii–xiii, 1–151.

3. Kmieć Z. Cooperation of liver cells in health and disease. *Adv Anat Embryol Cell Biol*. 2001; 161: iii–xiii, 1–151.

4. Kmieć Z. Cooperation of liver cells in health and disease. *Adv Anat Embryol Cell Biol*. 2001; 161: iii–xiii, 1–151.

5. Wang QM, Heinz BA. Recent advances in prevention and treatment of hepatitis C virus infections. In: Jucker E, ed. *Progress in Drug Research*. Vol. 55. Basel: Birkhäuser; 2001: 79–110.

6. Wang QM, Heinz BA. Recent advances in prevention and treatment of hepatitis C virus infections. In: Jucker E, ed. *Progress in Drug Research*. Vol. 55. Basel: Birkhäuser; 2001: 79–110.

7. Mondelli MU, Silini E. Clinical significance of hepatitis C virus genotypes. *J Hepatol*. 1999; 31(Suppl 1): 65–70.

8. Mondelli MU, Silini E. Clinical significance of hepatitis C virus genotypes. *J Hepatol*. 1999; 31(Suppl 1): 65–70.

9. Martinot-Peignoux M, Lapalus M, Asselah T, Marcellin P. The role of HBsAg quantification for monitoring natural history and treatment outcome. *Liver Int*. 2013; 33(Suppl 1):125--32; Li D, Gao G, Jiang H, Tang Z, Yu Y, Zang G. Hepatitis B virus-associated glomerulonephritis in HBsAg serological-negative patients. *Eur J Gastroenterol Hepatol*. 2015; 27(1): 65–69.

10. Martinot-Peignoux M, Lapalus M, Asselah T, Marcellin P. The role of HBsAg quantification for monitoring natural history and treatment outcome. *Liver Int*. 2013; 33(Suppl 1):125–32; Li D, Gao G, Jiang H, Tang Z, Yu Y, Zang G. Hepatitis B virus-associated glomerulonephritis in HBsAg serological-negative patients. *Eur J Gastroenterol Hepatol*. 2015; 27(1): 65–69.

11. McHutchison JG, Patel K. Future therapy of hepatitis C. *Hepatology*. 2002; 36(5 Suppl 1): S245–52.

12. Thio CL. Diagnosis, diagnostic tests and monitoring of hepatitis B virus in monoinfected and HIV-coinfected patients. *Antivir Ther*. 2007; McHutchison JG, Patel K. Future therapy of hepatitis C. *Hepatology*. 2002; 36(5 Suppl 1): S245–52.

13. McHutchison JG, Patel K. Future therapy of hepatitis C. *Hepatology*. 2002; 36(5 Suppl 1): S245–52.

14. Marnata C, Saulnier A, Mompelat D, et al. Determinants involved in hepatitis C virus and GB virus B primate host restriction. *J Virol.* 2015; 89(23): 12131–44; Marinho RT, Barreira DP. Hepatitis C, stigma and cure. *World J Gastroenterol*. 2013; 19(40): 6703–9.

15. Torok NJ, Dranoff JA, Schuppan D, Friedman SL. Strategies and endpoints of antifibrotic drug trials: Summary and recommendations from the AASLD Emerging Trends Conference, Chicago, June 2014. *Hepatology*. 2015; 62(2): 627–34.

16. Torok NJ, Dranoff JA, Schuppan D, Friedman SL. Strategies and endpoints of antifibrotic drug trials: Summary and recommendations from the AASLD Emerging Trends Conference, Chicago, June 2014. *Hepatology*. 2015; 62(2): 627–34.

28. COLLECTIVE EFFORTS

1. Tang N, Eisenberg JM, Meyer GS. The roles of government in improving health care quality and safety. *Jt Comm J Qual Saf*. 2004; 30(1): 47–55.

2. Ward JW. The hidden epidemic of hepatitis C virus infection in the United States: Occult transmission and burden of disease. *Top Antivir Med*. 2013; 21(1): 15–19.

3. Block TM, Alter HJ, London WT, Bray M. A historical perspective on the discovery and elucidation of the hepatitis B virus. *Antiviral Res*. 2016; 131: 109–23.

4. Sarbah SA, Younossi ZM. Hepatitis C: An update on the silent epidemic. *J Clin Gastroenterol*. 2000; 30(2): 125–43; Nelson KE, Shih JW, Zhang J, et al. Hepatitis E vaccine to prevent morbidity and mortality during epidemics. *Open Forum Infect Dis*. 2014; 1(3): ofu098.

5. Purtle J, Peters R, Brownson RC. A review of policy dissemination and implementation research funded by the National Institutes of Health, 2007–2014. *Implement Sci*. 2016; 11: 1.

6. Carcia J. Advancing quality improvement in public health. *Public Health Rep*. 2008; 123(6): 690–91; Field RI. Why is health care regulation so complex? *P T*. 2008 33(10): 607–8.

7. McDaniel PA, Malone RE. The role of corporate credibility in legitimizing disease promotion. *Am J Public Health*. 2009; 99(3): 452–61.

8. Connor BA, Patron DJ. Use of an accelerated immunization schedule for combined hepatitis A and B protection in the corporate traveler. *J Occup Environ Med*. 2008; 50(8): 945–50; Ibekwe RC, Ibeziako N. Hepatitis B vaccination status among health workers in Enugu, Nigeria. *Niger J Clin Pract*. 2006; 9(1): 7–10.

9. Lang EV. A better patient experience through better communication. *J Radiol Nurs*. 2012; 31(4): 114–19.

10. Scharer K. Internet social support for parents: The state of science. *J Child Adolesc Psychiatr Nurs*. 2005; 18(1): 26–35.

11. Chen TW. Paths toward hepatitis B immunization in South Korea and Taiwan. *Clin Exp Vaccine Res*. 2013; 2(2): 76–82.

12. Jessop AB, Cohen C, Burke MM, Conti M, Black M. Hepatitis support groups: Meeting the information and support needs of hepatitis patients. *Gastroenterol Nurs*. 2004; 27(4): 163–69; Cormier M. The role of hepatitis C support groups. *Gastroenterol Nurs*. 2005; 28(3 Suppl): S4–9.

29. HOPE, PATIENCE, CONFIDENCE, AND RESPONSIBILITY

1. Kylmä J, Duggleby W, Cooper D, Molander G. Hope in palliative care: An integrative review. *Palliat Support Care*. 2009; 7(3): 365–77.

2. Swisher AK. Patience and patients. *Cardiopulm Phys Ther J*. 2013; 24(2): 4.

3. Chen JY, Chung RT. Can we use the “C” word with confidence? Cure for chronic hepatitis C. *Gastroenterology*. 2011; 140(3): 766–68; Poovorawan Y, Sanpavat S, Pongpunglert W, et al. Long term efficacy of hepatitis B vaccine in infants born to hepatitis B e antigen-positive mothers. *Pediatr Infect Dis J*. 1992; 11(10): 816–21.

4. Coventry PA, Fisher L, Kenning C, Bee P, Bower P. Capacity, responsibility, and motivation: A critical qualitative evaluation of patient and practitioner views about barriers to self-management in people with multimorbidity. *BMC Health Serv Res*. 2014; 14: 536.

5. Ruiz ME. Risks of self-medication practices. *Curr Drug Saf*. 2010; 5(4): 315–23.

6. Kylmä J, Duggleby W, Cooper D, Molander G. Hope in palliative care: An integrative review. *Palliat Support Care*. 2009; 7(3): 365–77.

FURTHER READING

Askari F, Cutler D. *Hepatitis C, the Silent Epidemic: The Authoritative Guide*. New York: Perseus Books; 1999.

Bennett JE, Dolin R. *Latest Developments in Hepatitis* C. New York: Elsevier; 2015.

Blumberg BS. *Hepatitis B: The Hunt for a Killer Virus*. Princeton, NJ: Princeton University Press; 2002.

Carr BI. *Understanding Liver Cancer: A Tale of Two Diseases*. New York: Springer Healthcare; 2014.

Cohen MR, Gish RG, Doner K. *The Hepatitis C Help Book*. New York: St. Martin's Griffin; 2007.

Dickerson, JL. *Cirrhosis: An Essential Guide for the Newly Diagnosed*. New York: Da Capo Press; 2006.

Dolan M. *The Hepatitis C Handbook*. Berkley, CA: North Atlantic Books; 1999.

Hobbs C. *Natural Therapy for Your Liver*. New York: Avery; 2002.

Lawford CK, Sylvestre D. *Healing Hepatitis C*. New York; HarperCollins; 2009.

Palmer M. *Dr. Melissa Palmer's Guide to Hepatitis and Liver Disease*. New York: Avery; 2004.

Rains E. *Demon in My Blood: My Fight with Hep C—and a Miracle Cure*. Vancouver: Greystone Books; 2017.

Reau N, Jensen DM. *The New Hepatitis C: Effective Clinical Management in the Age of All-Oral Therapy*. Oxford: Oxford University Press; 2018.

Thuluvath PJ. *Hepatitis C: A Complete Guide for Patients and Families*. Baltimore: Johns Hopkins University Press; 2015.

Washington HA. *Living Healthy with Hepatitis C: Natural and Conventional Approaches to Recover Your Quality of Life*. New York: Dell; 2000.

INDEX

ABOUT THE AUTHOR

Naheed Ali, MD, PhD, began writing professionally in 2005. After completing lifestyle medicine training from Harvard Medical School in 2012, he graduated with a holistic health degree from elsewhere in 2013. His books can be found on the shelves in thousands of libraries across the globe. Visit him at http://naheedali.com.